ADVANCE PRAISE
FOR BEYOND RADIANT

"Marlyn Diaz has given us a masterpiece and a must read for any woman desiring to age well with beauty, happiness, and good health!"

> — Andrew Cohen, MD, FACS,
> Clinical Chief of Plastic Surgery Cedars-Sinai Hospital, Los Angeles

"A superfood and adaptogen adventure for body, mind, and spirit."

> — Julie Morris, Natural Food Chef, founder of Luminberry,
> and NYT best-selling author of six books,
> including *Superfood Smoothies*

"*Beyond Radiant* offers a perfect blueprint to help you achieve self-acceptance, the root of and route to health, happiness and success on your own terms."

> – David Allen, MD Integrative Medicine, Los Angeles, CA

"Marlyn is the 'Oprah' of Nutrition!"

> — Jennifer Skolnick, ESQ., Beverly Hills, CA

BEYOND
RADIANT

www.marlynwellness.com

Produced and printed by Tree of Life Books

Distributed by Tree of Life Books
Chief Editor and Muse: Joy E. Stocke
Cover Design: Jill Malek and Tim Ogline
Publication Design: Tim Ogline
Photographer: Jennifer Kelley
Makeup: Suzie Moldavon

Publisher's Cataloging-In-Publication Data
Diaz, Marlyn
Beyond Radiant: The Modern Woman's Guide to Health,
Healing, and Happiness in Midlife

ISBN: 978-1-7349563-2-0

Subjects: Health, Nutrition, Cooking, Lifestyle

Printed in the United States of America
First Edition

This book is intended to be a guidebook and reference volume only, not a medical manual. The information herewith has been researched to help you make informed decisions about your health and well-being, and it is not intended to be a substitute for any treatment that may have been prescribed by your doctor. If you suspect you have an issue with your health, please seek medical help.

The ideas, recipes, advice, and suggestions within the pages of this book are not intended as a substitute for a consultation with your physician. Neither the author nor the publisher shall be liable or responsible for any loss or damage allegedly arising from any information or suggestion in this book.

BEYOND RADIANT

THE MODERN WOMAN'S GUIDE TO HEALTH, HEALING, AND HAPPINESS IN MIDLIFE

MARLYN DIAZ, BSc Nutrition

Foreword by David Allen, MD

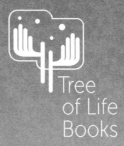

Tree
of Life
Books

CONTENTS

TO DANIEL AND JOSH,

my sons,

the light that I love.

May you always follow your hearts.

DEDICATED TO
YOU,
THE READER

I wrote this book for any woman ready to take her life higher. To reclaim her personal power while also understanding her body and how to feed it. It's for the woman who is tired. Tired of diets and to-do lists. Tired of trying to figure out how to feel better, have more energy, and look good in her sexy jeans too. It's for the woman who has reached a point where less feels like more. Where simple, clean, and whole sounds enticing and delicious. It's for the woman who is ready to take off her masks, the ones she has worn for so very, very long, and live from a place of honor, truth, peace, pleasure, righteousness, positivity, fulfillment, nourishment, and love. It's for the woman who is ready to say YES to HERSELF, and to all that she loves and enjoys.

If this is you, I welcome you. I'm so glad you're here. I honor you. I hear you. I see you. This book is dedicated to you. My wish is that it lights you up from the inside out and allows you to age gracefully with health and joy. I also hope it instills a deep love for caring for yourself and your body throughout the rest of your precious life.

WITH ALL MY LOVE,
Marlyn XOXO

FOREWORD

It is my great pleasure to introduce you to this magnificent book by nutritionist and lifestyle educator Marlyn Diaz. Since 2014, Marlyn and I have not only worked together (teaching workshops, supporting patients, and leading educational events), we've also become friends. Marlyn is the radiant woman she encourages women of all ages to embrace and become, especially in the second half of life.

Through our work separately and together, Marlyn and I know how hard it is to accept your inner radiance. Women are given unachievable models of what you should look like, be like, and act like. You are asked every day to face challenges and expectations. You're asked to maintain your careers while staying thin and beautiful. You are expected to be not only sensitive but also tough. You must be all things all the time to the people who rely on you. It's no wonder that I treat so many women suffering from depression, exhaustion, and other stress-related medical conditions.

Here's the good news. Marlyn has taken years of research and expertise and translated what she has learned and experienced into a book of miracles. *Beyond Radiant* offers a perfect blueprint to help you achieve self-acceptance, the root of and route to health, happiness, and success on your own terms. Follow Marlyn's positive, grounded, and gentle guidance and you will see miracles take place.

Marlyn is the friend who has been where you are, and she knows that miracles don't happen if you are constantly judging yourself harshly or comparing yourself to others in a negative light.

When you start where you are, the healing process can begin, enabling you to transform into your genuine fullness. With clear steps, dietary guidelines, and recipes made with fresh, beautiful food, Marlyn shows you how to begin where you are, create a plan, and embrace a lifestyle that allows you to become fully you.

Reaching midlife—defined as forty-plus—can present many challenges. At this point, many women feel stuck. Energy wanes, weight is easily gained and doesn't come off like before, hormones start fluctuating, sleep can become an issue, and we start losing our overall youthfulness.

Since most of us have the good chance of living to one hundred years old, now is the time to create our most radiant, healthy selves. We can transform our lives and health because there are very few obstacles that can't be overcome!

However, Marlyn knows what I have been telling patients for years: Your health will not be given to you in a doctor's office in the form of a pill. Marlyn's expertise about how our bodies work will not only enlighten you, it will also give you the tools you need to take responsibility for your health and learn how to optimize your body and mind. If you are someone who prioritizes others' needs over your own, you are not alone. If you have been relying on your good genes to get by, those good genes will only take you so far.

Which reminds me of a saying: "Up to forty, you have the face and body you got from your parents. After forty, you have the face and body you deserve."

Yes, transformation will take some work, some study, maybe some lifestyle changes, and asking for and getting help. And it can be done!

With Marlyn as your guide, I am excited about your journey ahead, because all the information you need is right here. Take your time and implement one idea at a time. As the Japanese concept of *kaizen* reminds us: small, ongoing, positive changes can reap major improvements.

So keep this book on your nightstand and read a little each night. Try one of Marlyn's Radiant Tips. Make one of her radiant shakes, or one of her delicious recipes, talk to your friends about all you're learning and consider forming a group to support each other in the process.

I wish you good and radiant luck on your journey with my friend Marlyn!

– David R. Allen, MD
Integrative Medicine
Los Angeles, 2020

YOUR WELLNESS ROADMAP

- Better health

- More energy

- Greater joy

- Sharper focus

- Less brain fog

- Healthier moods

- More fulfilling sex life

- Deeper sleep

- Happier relationships

- Increased self-confidence

- An awakening of dreams

- Living life with more passion, purpose, and pleasure

Throughout these pages, we'll take a journey together—a journey of health, wellness, beauty, and love. I'm excited to be your guide. As we walk together, I'll share my secrets, strategies, wisdom, and tried-and-true ways to become your most vibrant, energetic, healthiest self—the best possible version of YOU. I'll take you on a health food store tour and show you the ins and outs of the latest healthy foods: things to buy and those to avoid. I'll meet you in your kitchen and assist you in purging your pantry and filling it up with exciting new superfoods, adaptogens, and satisfying treats. I'll sit down with you at your favorite restaurant, look over the menu, and guide you through making healthy choices, so you know just the things to order to keep your mind sharp and your figure fit. I'll spend time with you before you head off to vacation or to the beach, so you know just what to pack for a fun-filled, immune-boosting trip. I'll even share my favorite recipes and give you simple cooking tips I've learned from accomplished chefs along the way.

My greatest intent is to empower you, so wherever you are, wherever you go, you will have the tools to become the vibrant, joy-filled, radiant woman you were meant to be. And here's some more good news: I'm going to make this journey sexy, fun, and simple. All you have to do is show up and join me with your biggest, most curious self, an open heart and mind, and a willingness to look at your eating, exercise, sleep, self-care, and lifestyle patterns with a new eye and a new perspective. You can try on what you want, incorporate what you like, and leave the rest behind. Or, you can dive in and shift it all at once. The choice is up to you.

As Glinda the Good Witch said to Dorothy in *The Wizard of Oz*, "You've always had the power, my dear." My desire is to shed some light, make our journey fun, and help you rediscover your own inner power—the one that's been there all along. So let's get started with a session in my office to get acquainted. Come on in, pull up a seat, and join me. I'm so glad you're here.

INTRODUCTION

"YOU GOTTA CHANGE!"

In June 2017, I sat in the front row of a small theater in Maria Shriver's corporate office on San Vicente Boulevard for her live interview series, "Architects of Change." That evening, Maria was conducting her last interview of the season. It featured transgender writer, producer, and actress Janet Mock, who was there to promote her new book, *Surpassing Certainty.*

I had tried to attend one of Maria's earlier interviews to no avail and had not been aware of Janet Mock. But if Maria was interviewing her, I reasoned, I wanted to be there.

As a certified nutritionist and wellness coach, I attend yearly medical conferences, nutrition workshops, health food shows, and lectures. I've long been a fan and admirer of Maria Shriver, journalist, author, and former First Lady of California. I've watched the eloquent way she has handled adversity in the face of personal loss and betrayal. The people she attracts and her beauty inside and out captivated me then and inspire me now.

On the day Maria interviewed Janet, I should have been on top of the world. I had a growing list of clients whom I loved and respected, many in midlife, seeking transformation through better health. At the same time, I was going through some pretty heavy sh*t myself. I had recently been diagnosed with stage 1 breast cancer. On top of that, after twenty years of marriage, my husband and I were going through a separation, leaving me worried about an uncertain financial future. My husband and I were still living in the same home with our two boys and I was trying my best to remain positive.

The good news is that after minor surgery, I remain in remission. And, after years of tough conversations, letting go of anger and resentment, and a continued effort to show up in kindness and love, my ex and I have worked through our "stuff" and have become peaceful friends and better co-parenting partners. Day by day, I strive to control what I can, which means that I follow the advice I tailor for my clients by buying and preparing foods that nourish and heal my body, by actively engaging with people and activities that inspire me, and by knowing how I act and think today will build a better tomorrow.

Truth is: To achieve our goals, we all need those souls we can rely on and trust. I strive to be a nurturing, supportive soul for the extraordinary people I counsel, to share my gifts and provide warmth, connection, and sisterhood. Whether you are a client in my private practice or have attended one of my workshops, online programs, or events, you are part of a larger community, one in which we lift each other up.

When arriving at a crossroad, I've come to understand that each decision made in that moment is an opportunity for me—and for you—to renew the story of our lives.

Each and every one of my clients has arrived at their own crossroads. Many have gone through adversity or hard times. I help them get to the root of what is blocking their path, which means building their healthiest, strongest bodies. I've learned that hidden roots and underlying issues, like chronic inflammation, out-of-whack hormones, and ongoing pain, can block us from losing weight, feeling great about ourselves, and overcoming addictive behaviors.

Speaking of which, I know how easy it is to go for the quick fix—that extra slice of pizza, order of curly fries, or pint of creamy, mint-chocolate-chip ice cream. I've been there. There are reasons for our cravings for fat, sugar, and carbs. Those calorie-dense foods create endorphins signaling to our brains that all is peaceful and well. That endorphin rush of sugar and carbs hits the part of the brain responsible for pleasure in the same way sex and some drugs do. Consuming sugar and certain foods stimulates the release of dopamine, a neurotransmitter that gives us a sense of euphoria, leading our bodies to immediately feel better. Thus, the cycle of craving and reward repeats itself until we say "enough," or until our bodies break down.

In addition to eating foods that nourish us, this same chemical rush can be found in healthier ways of living. A loving hug, a night out with the girls, or being of service to another releases a tide of oxytocin. Even the simple act of holding the door open for someone or smiling at a stranger or, heaven forbid, letting a car in front of you on the crowded LA freeway sets those chemicals in motion. Your reward? A hormonal high, or that feel-good sensation we know so well after finishing that pint of ice cream. It's all here for our pleasure.

Through thousands of conversations I've had over the years, I've been privy to a lot of personal revelations from clients, audiences at my lectures, and participants in my online programs. Challenges I've noticed that keep people from a healthy lifestyle include early childhood trauma, financial issues, marriage challenges, relationship upsets, career stress, children at various stages of development, and so much more. Many of these challenges lead to unhealthy eating patterns, which only make us feel worse. We don't believe we deserve what we desire. And we ask ourselves, "Do I really deserve to have the body, relationships, financial wherewithal, and, ultimately, the life I desire?"

I say, why not feel beautiful? Why not take a few moments and eat some delicious, mouth-watering pink watermelon, or sweet, juicy figs with almond butter, or roasted sweet potatoes and yams (which naturally contain over 50 percent of our daily requirement for vitamin C and help women stimulate the production of progesterone in the ovaries, the calming hormone we begin to lose in our forties)? A rainbow of colors and a combination of healthy fats, protein, and fiber are what our body truly craves to feel good and in balance.

As a nutritionist, wellness coach, and business owner, I'm also a cheerleader, an educator, and, as many clients tell me, a healer. You could call me a wounded healer. Because in dealing with my own adversity, I draw great strength from people who share their stories with me, who have moved through their own challenges and, who, one step at a time, have walked into healthier, stronger bodies, and—YES! — have become equally empowered to engage fully in life.

The question we must ask ourselves is this: Will I carry adversities with me, or let them go?

With patience, intestinal fortitude (literally making our guts happy), and a willingness to stay with the process—even when we get knocked down—the answer, again, is YES! And, believe me, I know, because I also know what it feels like to be that cartoon punching bag, knocked down over and over, only to rise back up.

If you're reading this, chances are you've been there too. And welcome to the human race.

That's where I come in to help you rebuild your body (and mind) by showing you the foods and lifestyle habits that will strengthen you. I will train you in habits and simple techniques that will allow you to feel your best, look your best, and age your best—with the goal of optimal health and radiant well-being at your core. Just the mere fact of starting your day with a glass of water, into which you've added fresh lemon juice, helps eliminate waste and cleanses your liver (the oil filter of the body). Or beginning with a smoothie loaded with energizing superfoods like raw cacao (mood boosting), matcha green tea (immune and metabolism boosting), or pearl powder (beauty boosting because it naturally contains lots of readily available collagen, calcium, and minerals, which we lose as we age) can lay the foundation for a day filled with energy, stamina, and pure radiance as opposed to a day filled with dread and drab.

Clients come to me with health issues. Weight challenges. Food challenges. Some feel shame, some remorse. Most are unsure how to get to where they want to go. So we sit. And we talk. And we look at it all. With love and light and understanding. And from there, we decide, we are here. Let's create a roadmap to move forward.

Which brings me back to Maria Shriver and Janet Mock. Magic happens when we're in the presence of empowered women who have stepped into their truth. It's not that they, or we, are perfect. It's the fact that powerful women are willing to be vulnerable and authentic. Sitting in the audience that evening, I recognized that I too could not only *be* empowered, I was *already* powerful, just as I was. I was lucky to be in the embrace of the collective energy of Janet and Maria and a community of women (and others) who were there to grow with me. Together, we were forming the ground of being for healing.

During Janet and Maria's conversation, it became clear that at times we as women lose our voices. In my work, I've seen how this has been carried forward for generations. When we lose our voices, we lose our power. And the accepted solution for many of us when there is nowhere else to turn is to eat the wrong foods and drink one too many glasses of wine.

But there was Janet, sharing her story about how, with the support of friends and family, she began her transition from a male body to a female body in her teens. How she became the first in her family to attend college. She would go on to build a successful career in journalism and currently writes for and stars in the Netflix series *Pose*. But what hit me was how, at twenty-nine, Janet made the decision to become her most authentic, powerful, truest self, entering her thirties with a newfound freedom and personal strength.

At the end of the interview Maria opened up the floor for questions. I immediately raised my hand and asked Janet, "How did you get the confidence to become your most authentic self at twenty-nine? I'm in my fifties and I still feel like there's a part of me hiding out. And what advice do you have for us to show up fully without dying with our music inside?"

Janet's reply echoed the work I do with my clients. "Be uncertain," she said, flashing her beautiful smile. "There's no linear path. Start by making little decisions each day to be yourself. Be willing to look at the relationships that are holding you back in some way. Really see if some of those relationships are productive for you to be in. Speaking out and being yourself is also going to require some sacrifices. You're going to have to shed some people, shed some relationships, shed some ways in which you have done things [routines], things that make you feel comfortable."

Bravo, I thought. So many times when someone is trying to lose weight, they tell me that they want to shed the extra pounds. But without shedding ingrained habits—and frankly, a distorted view of their gorgeous selves—they can't find the way through to truly embody the body they already have.

I could see Maria nodding. "You gotta change!" She paused, grew thoughtful, and added, "And that's hard."

The moment Maria shared those strong and poignant words—"You gotta change"—something inside of me, already in motion, shifted. I left determined to take courageous action steps over the next few days and months. It made me remember that we *all* have the power to change at any moment. It takes a decision and desire to do things differently. It may be hard at times, it will be uncomfortable, and it will be different than anything else we have ever done. But at the same time, it can be incredibly exciting, rewarding, confidence-building, adventurous, and fun. I'm here to vouch for that.

The thing is, I was the one who showed up that evening to listen to a profound conversation. Janet and Maria's message came through at the right time because I was the one who wanted to change.

And here I am, a voice for you, with all the wisdom and practical knowledge I've earned. I'm here to take a stand for your greatest health and wellness—from the inside out. To support you in reclaiming your voice and your confidence. To give you permission to drop the old limiting beliefs and stories and become the greatest version of you.

Are you ready?

Let's go!

PART I:

KNOWLEDGE
IS POWER

Chapter 1

THE RADIANT WOMAN

And the day came when the risk to remain tight in
a bud was more painful than the risk it took to blossom.

– A N A Ï S   N I N

THE HEROINE'S JOURNEY

Rewind to the seventies. My journey in nutrition began in 1978 when I wrote my first high school term paper on food additives and their effect on the body. You could say that I was ahead of my time. There was no Dr. Oz or many other health influencers filling the pages of magazines, and there were no blog sites to troll in the middle of the night. And all those popular magazines like *Seventeen* featured fad diets. While it was the beginning of the health food era, it was also the era of cooking convenience food and bringing home Fritos, Cheetos, and Cap'n Crunch.

I recall going out to Chinese dinners with my family, eating pork fried rice, chicken chow mein, and fried wonton noodles dipped in duck sauce, and beginning to notice that the food was giving me headaches. I started tracing it back to the MSG. You could say it was an aha moment, or my first connection and realization that the food I ate had a direct effect on how I felt.

My passion for food and nutrition, then and now, is based on wanting to feel better, look better, and *be* better. Back then, I was constantly searching for quick fixes so that I could fit into my bell-bottom, hip-hugger Jordache jeans and be healthy and happy. I instinctively knew there was another way, though at the time I didn't have all the pieces to the health puzzle.

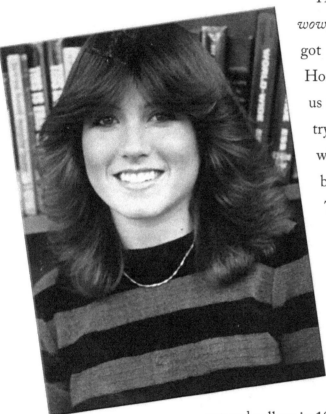

Here I am, forty years ago! Holy *wow*, how time flies. This picture got me elected as my high school's Homecoming Queen! But like most of us at that age, inside I was struggling, trying to find myself and understand who I was. I ate *a lot* of carbs and sugar back then too. I loved Chips Ahoy!, Tastykakes (that's the Philly girl in me), and Dairy Queen vanilla ice cream cones dipped in sprinkles. (Oh, and I smoked cigarettes to be cool.) Yet I was always on the search for the magic key to wellness and weight loss.

That's a big reason why, when I entered college in 1980, I decided to study nutrition and food science. It's taken me years to find the answers. Decades to understand myself and how to effectively nourish a body and a mind. And it's taken a lot of growing, forgiving, and letting go. I honor this girl for all that she's been through—and how she keeps *showing up* fully no matter what. I love that she's found so many of the answers she was seeking, and how she's created a life where she's deeply devoted to helping others—especially women—find their nutrition and wellness answers too.

One could say my nutrition journey has been a calling.

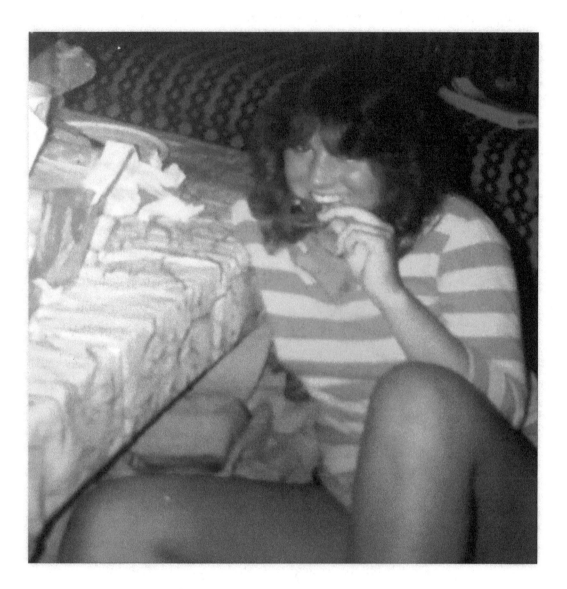

Me at twenty, in college studying nutrition. Struggling inside.
Eating chocolate-covered pretzels and potato chips—
a great salty/sweet, crunchy combo!

I'm now at this place called midlife, a far cry from that teenage girl searching for the answers and the keys to glowing health and well-being. I've learned how to cultivate radiance from within and am always researching new ways to stay healthy, fit, and happy.

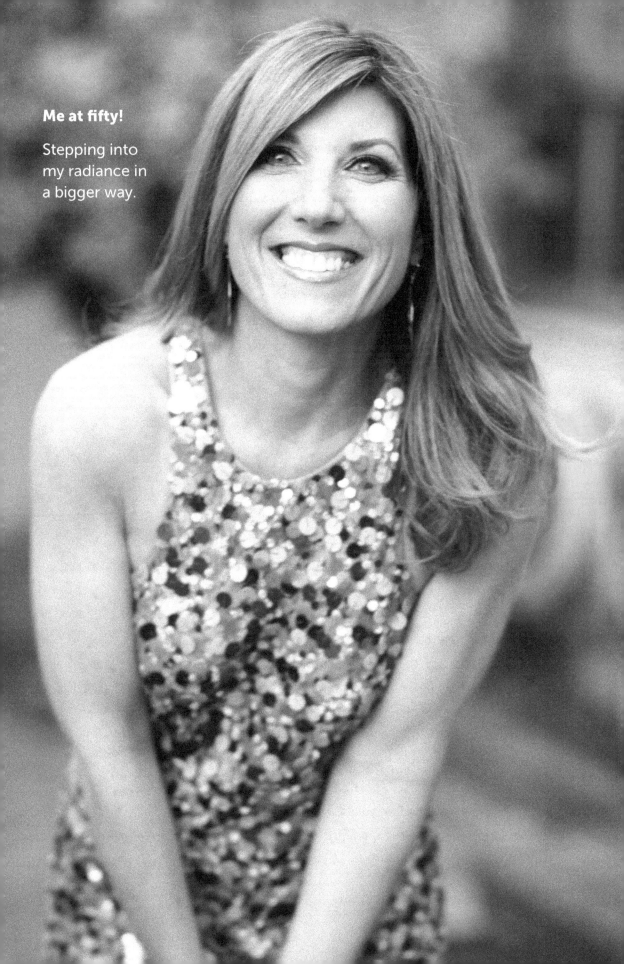

Me at fifty!

Stepping into
my radiance in
a bigger way.

WELLNESS IS AN INSIDE JOB

I've come to realize that wellness is an inside job. I've learned through research, and through my own life experience, that certain principles work. They may have to be modified at times. But they are sound principles that have the potential to take us into old age—principles that can carry us forward into every new chapter of our lives through our forties, fifties, sixties, and beyond.

Truth is, if we're radiant in midlife, if we pay attention to our mindsets plus our diets, we will have an easier time moving through the aging process. And when we pay attention to what our bodies are trying to tell us, we'll become more in tune with our truth as well. My truth might look different from your truth, though what I believe most of us truly want is to look and feel radiant every day of our lives. I know I do. My clients do. How about you?

There's no time like the present to choose into wellness.

So, let's begin.

WE BECOME RADIANT
ONE DAY AT A TIME

By the time we reach our midlife years, we've lived a lot of life. Many of us are exhausted, frustrated, or unclear of our next steps. Maybe you've been raising kids, working super hard at your career or business, or maybe you've been struck with an unforeseen health challenge, death of a partner or loved one, or have to care for an aging parent or sick child. Or maybe you got divorced, or have hit a really hard financial crisis along the way.

We don't plan for these events. Sometimes they just happen like a big fat BOOM! You wake up one day and say, "Wait a second here. This isn't what I had pictured for my life. This isn't the way things were supposed to turn out."

And lo and behold, they did. And then what? You can sit and fret and wish and cry—and sometimes that is JUST what is needed.

But someday it may hit you that you still have time. Time to change things. Time to let go and use it all for your highest growth and learning. What I've come to know for sure is that our life experience and challenging life moments are always an opportunity for our highest growth and learning. Even the tough, yucky stuff.

When life gets messy—which it will—give yourself permission to live again and to love again. Give yourself permission to fall down and get back up. This is growth.

One of my biggest learnings and greatest gifts to myself and to my clients has been this: "Be your own mother" (or father). That's self-care. That's growing up. Mature love. Loving yourself like you wish your mother or father (or caretaker) would/did. YOU can do this. It's healing work. It may be tough at times, and you're worth it!

WHAT DOES A RADIANT WOMAN LOOK LIKE?

She's fresh. She's fierce. She's fabulous. She has glowing skin, a beautiful smile, a skip in her step, and a body and mind that says YES I can.

She radiates beauty, health, love, and positivity. She lives in joy, abundance, prosperity, and possibility. She knows who she is and she knows where she wants to go. Even when she meets with an obstacle or roadblock, she is guided by the governing principle: Where there's a will there's a way.

The radiant woman is courageous and bold and takes care of herself. She unapologetically loves her life. She shines her light bright and fills her cup with loving acts of kindness and radical self-care.

Is she perfect? No.

Is her life messy at times? Yes.

Is she an ever-blossoming work in progress? You betcha!

And here's the thing too.

She's immensely clear that her health and well-being are first on her priority list, because without them, she's lost. She nourishes herself from the inside out and the outside in. Healthy food is her fuel and loving acts of kindness are her refuge.

HAVE YOU LOST YOUR RADIANCE? OR PART OF IT?

Losing your radiance may look something like this: You're tired, spent, exhausted, and deeply wanting to feel better again. Your weight is slowly rising, your doctor is unhappy with the results of your latest blood tests, and the clothes in your closet no longer fit.

If you feel like you've lost your glow, I will help you find your way back to health. With a couple of simple tweaks and a few new habits, you can crowd out the chemicals, ignite your metabolism, heal your nervous system, and step into your million-dollar self.

The majority of the women I work with are successful, educated, and smart. Yet when it comes to their middle-aged bodies and changing health, they are lost. Most are extremely stressed and addicted to high amounts of coffee, sugar, and carbs during the day and are using comfort foods like bread, cheese, chocolate, and wine during the evenings and weekends to calm down. (Yes, there is a place in your diet for your favorite foods and drinks. What it comes down to is when, why, and how much, and how you incorporate them. More on that in the coming chapters.) For now, I want you to know that when you're eating out of stress or an addiction to certain foods, it can lead to a vicious cycle of blood sugar highs and lows, weight gain, and an incredibly stressed-out nervous system with accompanying lack of energy and low stamina.

"Food is the enemy!"

"Keto, paleo, vegan!
I'm completely overwhelmed and confused."

"Menopause sucks! I seriously cannot lose weight. I'm just frustrated."

These are the types of things I hear from women all the time. When we first get to talking, I inevitably discover that most are completely confused with all of the diet and nutrition information available today. They've tried to get back on track with the old high-protein, low-carb regimens, calorie-restricted food delivery programs, or juice cleanse plans. And guess what? They've failed. Many times over. Additionally, the majority of women I see and talk with take medications for everything from depression, anxiety, acid indigestion, high cholesterol count, high blood sugar, and low thyroid.

Their doctors have prescribed them a pill for the symptoms instead of a solution for the cause.

That's where my revolutionary work comes in. When you understand the relationship between food and health and how to change the composition of what you eat and how you live, you can begin to gain back control of your mind, mood, energy, and body.

CINDY'S STORY:
THE ART OF TAKING BACK CONTROL

Cindy, a petite, fifty-seven-year-young woman living in Los Angeles and the mother of four grown children, reached out after hearing me speak at a women's wellness conference. Cindy spent most of her life trying to eat healthy foods and care for herself. After going through menopause, she was finding it extremely challenging to lose weight and maintain a body she was happy in. She found herself eating more food than she was used to and choosing things that were not always in the best interest of her highest health and well-being. Along with her weight challenges, she was experiencing sleepless nights, intense sugar cravings, hormonal fluctuations, and exhaustion.

Cindy needed a reset, so together we decided that she would embark on my 21-day transformational food cleanse plan, which included crowding out pro-inflammatory foods like gluten, dairy, processed soy, refined sugars, and industrial oils. I also added in a few key supplements: alpha-lipoic acid, berberine, chromium, and L-carnitine, specifically designed to target her sugar cravings, sluggish metabolism, and fatigue. After three months, Cindy lost eight pounds, had more energy, fewer sugar cravings, greater consciousness around her food choices, and more restful sleep. As a huge bonus, her husband of forty years followed the plan alongside her and lost ten pounds. Our biweekly and regular email sessions helped keep Cindy accountable and on track.

At the end of our coaching journey, Cindy shared her biggest takeaway: "This new way of eating and living is so freeing.

The part I love best is being completely comfortable with, rather than obsessed by, food and my body. Keeping it simple made it easy and doable. I was so out of control. To finally have control is such a powerful feeling!"

THE RADIANT TEEN AND YOUNG ADULT

The basic principles throughout this book work for all ages. Eating well and living well is a practice. Go ahead and share these principles and healthy practices with your daughters and sons, especially those in their teens and twenties. As we create our health and wellness plan, we are helping our children set themselves up with healthy practices and delicious ways of eating, so they can live vibrantly throughout their lives.

TRUST THE PROCESS

"The day you plant the seed is not the day
you eat the fruit."

To initiate change, we must drop the stories that hold us back. The stories that keep us stuck, safe, and living small. The stories we've been telling ourselves for so very long. They may sound something like, "I'm not good enough. I'm so frustrated. I can't do this. I failed so many times before. Who am I to deserve what I truly want?"

Or perhaps your stories are made up of the wounds and anger you still hold for your mother, father, ex, or childhood friend. Stories come in different shapes and forms. Most of us keep them locked away until one day we wake up and realize these stories and old ways of being no longer serve us. They keep us from growing into our most vibrant, healthy selves. When these old stories come up, we may find that we grip, clutch, and hold on tight because, "Who would we be without them?"

What stories of the past are you still carrying that are defining the you of today?

Are you creating your life, or are you a victim of it?

Wherever you go, you are creating you. We spend so much time clutching, holding, striving, and gripping the parts of ourselves from yesteryear. Imagine if you were to let go. Imagine if you knew you were highly supported. Imagine if you were to allow your body to relax, unwind, and come down from its highly addictive stress levels. Who could you be?

I know this firsthand. For the most part, it's been hard for me to talk about challenges in my life. Keeping it all "safe" inside led me to high states of stress, bouts of shame, and a feeling of less than—which in turn led to hiding out, isolation, and emotional eating.

I felt myself playing small and keeping the best parts of me locked away. What helped move me forward was making a decision to join a women's group in 2009, led by two extraordinary coaches: Carolyn Freyer-Jones and Michelle Bauman. Carolyn and Michelle gave me a new perspective on the power of community and the value of sharing the intimate moments of our lives with other supportive women in a safe and loving environment. During that time, my nutrition coaching business was born. When I began to pay close attention, I realized the times I felt my very best and brightest were the times I was coaching clients. By helping a client shift their life for the better, I was able to get out of my head and into my heart and build a bigger life than I ever dreamed possible.

LISA'S JOURNEY:
RELEASING ANGER AND LOSING WEIGHT

At sixty-two, successful, beautiful, and highly educated, Lisa was living with a lot of anger toward her mother. In a eureka moment, she realized some of this anger had carried forward from her early childhood years. Wanting to stay on the good side of her mother, she put up with unreasonable demands and tolerated behaviors that she would never have tolerated from anyone else. This way of being drove her stress levels through the roof. As a result, her body was unable to relax, release weight, and feel its best. Honestly, Lisa was flat-out exhausted.

Despite changing the food she ate and creating new ways of living, moving, and sleeping, she was having a tough time releasing the weight she wanted to lose. During one of our coaching sessions, and after weeks of following my 21-day transformational food cleanse, she decided it was time to own her part in her story and discuss this with her mother.

Within days of sharing her truth and stating that she would no longer tolerate disrespect, Lisa put her own loving boundaries in place and began making new decisions regarding her relationship with her mother and also with others in her life. In the next few weeks, Lisa's stress levels began to lessen, her weight slowly started to come off, and her new food plan was finally taking shape.

Lisa continues to integrate her healthy habits and nourishing lifestyle rituals into her life and now feels better than she has in years.

I share Lisa's story as an example and an invitation to become more conscious in your own life of how events and emotions may be affecting you. Everything is energy—even your thoughts. Thoughts create reality. Thoughts can inhibit our goals and dreams. Thoughts can also move them forward. I invite you to take a moment throughout your day to become more conscious of your thoughts. Become aware of your awareness. Get curious. Notice where your thoughts lead you and what they have to say. Also, take a look at who or what is pulling you out of alignment. Who or what is depleting you. It could be a person, food, habit, or something in your environment. It may take some slowing down and really observing your life from a new point of view. Stay with it, I promise you it's worth it—and so are you.

THE POWER OF MIDLIFE

Midlife is a time of awakening. Midlife is a time to stop, pause, and pivot.

Speaking of pivoting, before we move forward, let's take a moment to make a calming cup of herbal tea.

Perhaps you enjoy chamomile, mint, or my favorite, rooibos. Preparing and drinking a cup of tea is a lovely ritual and a beautiful way to relax, unwind, and calm down from the busy-ness of the day.

And while we're at it, let's focus on our breath. Take a long, slow, deep breath. Let it in and slowly let it out. And once more—deeply inhale and fill your gorgeous lungs with lots of fresh air and oxygen, and slowly exhale. Aaaahhhhh.

Deep breathing and herbal tea breaks are a wonderful way to reduce stress, nourish our bodies, and soothe our spirits, any time of day or night.

Okay, let's continue…

MIDLIFE WILL ASK YOU TO:

- Do things you've never done before.
- Love your body, even as it goes through radical changes and shifts.
- Get quiet, go inside, and listen deeply.
- Shed the veils and masks you've been wearing for so long.
- Become more vulnerable, courageous, and bold.

Midlife is a time for women to slow down and ask for what they want and need. Our bodies are transforming before our eyes, energetically and physically. We have to reimagine our lives, redefine beauty, change our relationship with the things we've always known to be true, and revise our health as well.

And here's the good news: At any moment you can change.

YOU CAN…

- Choose into health. Choose into more confidence.
- Choose into your strengths. Choose into living through the best parts of you.

YOU CAN ALSO GIVE YOURSELF PERMISSION TO...

- Let go of your old stories *(this is a biggie!!)*.
- Get clear on what you want and need.
- Let go of the people, places, and things that are no longer serving you or no longer bring you joy.
- Love deeper.

STAY IN THE COMPANY OF WELLNESS

Look around at the women in your life. Whom do you admire? Why?

It can be a powerful exercise to slow down, get curious, and seek out women we admire most for their healthy habits and positive empowering lifestyle traits. It actually gives the brain proof of what's possible.

STEP INTO YOUR RADIANCE WITH COMMITMENT

Stepping into your radiance and owning it is part of your ongoing commitment to your life's journey. Your story is unique, though the core premise of caring for yourself and becoming the best version of you at all stages of life will remain the foundation for our work together and for your own aging process.

The chapters ahead will provide you with tools that you'll use daily. For now, I'm sharing my recipe for the Beyond Radiant smoothie. This simple and delicious smoothie can be a beautiful part of your day and week. Give it a try.

THE BEYOND RADIANT SMOOTHIE

Based on the Beyond Radiant food principles of combining protein, fat, and fiber, the Beyond Radiant Smoothie is a delightful part of my proprietary 21-day transformational food cleanse. (More about that in Chapter 9.)

The Beyond Radiant Smoothie includes a very special ingredient, a fruit called amla berry, also known as the Indian gooseberry. Amla berry has been used in Ayurvedic (Indian) medicine for thousands of years to boost immunity and improve health.

Its central properties help fight off cell aging (free radical damage) and cell degeneration.

Amla is one of the highest and most potent sources of antioxidants on planet Earth, and it is loaded with vitamin A and vitamin C (eight times more vitamin C than an orange), plus it's brimming with cancer-kicking antioxidants, polyphonols, flavonoids, and alkaloids.

Research shows amla can help boost metabolism, reduce blood sugar levels (due to its high chromium content), stave off cravings, build immunity, beautify hair and skin, reduce inflammation, improve heart health, and promote eye health too.

Note: Suggested serving is no more than ½ to 1 teaspoon each day.

THE BEYOND RADIANT SMOOTHIE
INGREDIENTS:

- 1 cup unsweetened almond milk, or other plant-based milk
- ½ cup berries (organic blueberries, strawberries, or mixed); fresh or frozen
- 1 tablespoon ground flaxseed, organic
- 1 heaping teaspoon almond butter, organic
- 1 teaspoon MCT oil*
- 1 scoop plant-based protein powder
- 1 teaspoon of amla powder, organic

OPTIONAL BEAUTY ADD-INS:

- 1 teaspoon matcha green tea powder (metabolism booster)
- 1 teaspoon raw cacao powder (mood booster)
- 1 handful spinach (blood cleanser, beauty enhancer)

Place almond milk, berries, ground flaxseed, almond butter, MCT oil, protein powder, and amla powder in a blender. On a medium-high setting, blend until combined and frothy, 1 to 2 minutes. Or, before blending, add the optional matcha green tea powder, raw cacao powder, and/or spinach.

Pour, sip, and *enjoy*.

*NOTE: **About MCT and why I like it for this recipe.** MCT oil is made up of medium chain triglyceride fats found in coconut oil. MCT oil supports weight loss and enhances endurance during workouts. Unlike long chain triglycerides that take time to be utilized as energy, MCT goes straight to the liver and is used as a quick source of energy. MCT oil also promotes the release of leptin, called "the feel-full hormone." (More about leptin in Chapter 3.)

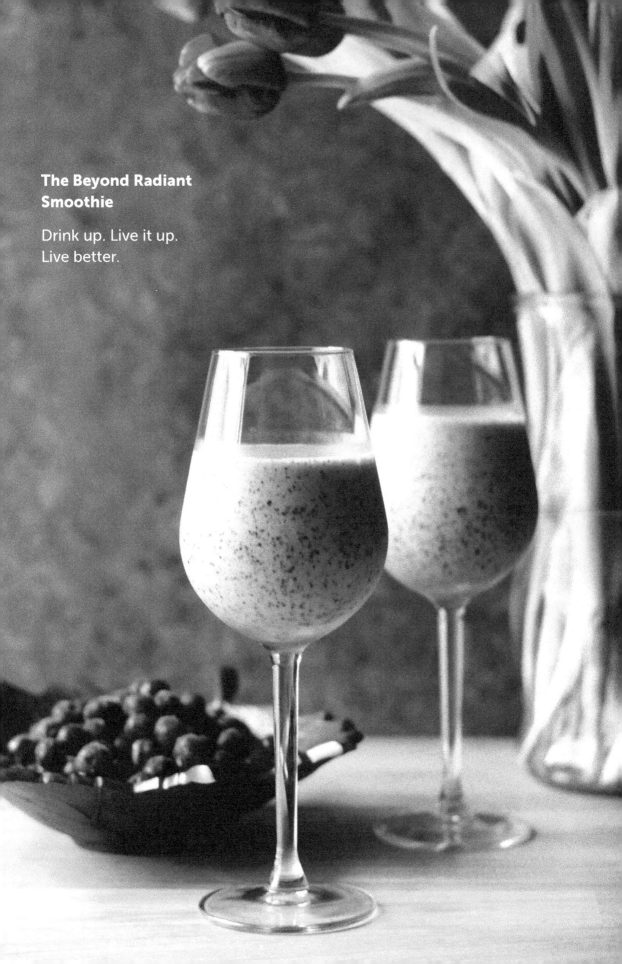

The Beyond Radiant Smoothie

Drink up. Live it up.
Live better.

Chapter 2

THE 3 C'S: CLARITY, COURAGE, AND COMMITMENT

The path to success starts with three words: clarity, courage, and commitment.

1. The **clarity** to know the old paradigm is no longer working and that change is in order.
2. The **courage** to take that step forward and do things differently.
3. The **commitment** to stick with your plan.

I've worked with hundreds of clients over the last decade plus, and I've seen it all: success, failure, frustration, and resolution. Some clients are relentless in their approach to eating better and taking back their health. Some are passive. And others are somewhere in the middle.

What makes one person successful while another slips back into their old ways?

A desire to change, the boldness to do it, and a willingness to take each day as it comes.

Most clients call me because they want change. Their desire for change happens for a reason: a health scare, an uncomfortable feeling, a spiritual awakening, or a deep-rooted unpleasant emotion that gnaws at them daily.

What I've learned is this: If we ignore or resist what bothers us, it will persist and resurface again and again.

WHAT ABOUT YOU?

WHY DO YOU WANT TO MAKE A CHANGE?

SOME ANSWERS I HEAR INCLUDE:

"I feel stuck, stressed out, and my skin has lost its glow."

"My clothes are not fitting and I feel awful in my body."

"I'm on multiple medications for various conditions and I want to get off the meds."

"My blood tests are showing less than optimal numbers."

"I have no energy. I feel like a slug."

"I'm back in the dating scene and I want to look my best."

THE QUESTIONS I ASK IN RETURN:

"Are you ready to make a commitment to yourself and do things differently than you have in the past to create the future you desire?"

"Are you willing to stick with your plan and be in it for the long game, even when you fall?"

LET'S BREAK DOWN THE THREE C'S AND LOOK AT EACH BRIEFLY.

CLARITY

At our first meeting, most clients say to me, "I want to feel better."

Their weight is up, their energy is down, their sleep is off, and usually high stress levels are at play. All this leads to a cascade of events in the body. And that's exactly where clarity and inspiration come from. You've made the call and are ready to act, to do things differently. When my clients and I meet, I have them fill out a short health history questionnaire.

The form starts with simple questions that lead to profound insight:

"Are you waking in the night? If so, what time?"

"Are you on medications?"

"What are you eating for breakfast, lunch, and dinner?"

"Do you currently have any health challenges?"

"What is the health history of your parents?"

And finally, "Where do you want to go from here?"

As we go through the answers, a broader picture begins to emerge for both of us.

Most women I work with want to have enough energy so they can live a great life full of joy and happiness. Most want to go through the day without needing lots of caffeine, sugar, and alcohol. Most want to have enough stamina to work out, run their errands, create their business deals, and enjoy their families and friends while looking good and aging well. As they build a better body, most clients challenge those around them to get healthy too—often at great benefit to all of those in their lives.

Once *you* get clear and are ready to make a change, we can begin looking at the food you eat, your lifestyle habits, your medications, your environment, your sleep, and the biggest area, your stress. Stress often leads to physical and psychological changes that can have long-lasting side effects.

Ongoing stress sets off a series of reactions in the body that contribute to anxiety, tension, sleepless nights, irritability, and inflammation.

Stress is one of the biggest driving factors in poor health and weight gain. It can affect the body in ways that are difficult to see from the outside. It can lead to emotional eating, high blood pressure, low thyroid, high blood sugar, belly fat, and so much more. This in turn can all lead to weight gain, low energy, and hormonal imbalances.

It's also important to be aware that we can become addicted to our stress. Think about the act of worrying. When we continuously worry about things, we set our bodies up to produce high amounts of cortisol. (I will talk more about cortisol in Chapter 3.) High amounts of cortisol, produced over time can make you fat, age you faster, contribute to an inflamed body, and wreak havoc on your health. The first step to end this unhealthy cycle is to become aware of your relationship to your stress.

What positive action steps do you take when you get stressed? Do you work out? Practice deep breathing? Go for a walk?

What unhealthy action steps do you find yourself immersed in when you're stressed? Do you grab the carton of ice cream? Down a Snickers bar? Yell at the dog?

Take time to notice all the ways in which you relate to your stress.

In the next few chapters, I present a clear roadmap and some basic concepts so we can become more empowered to gain control over our circumstances. We'll also gain a clear understanding of the interrelationship between our food, blood, health, and stress, and how it all relates to inflammation, disease, and weight gain. **Knowledge is indeed power!**

Once you see how all the dots connect, it not only becomes easier to shift your habits and implement new healthier routines, it also becomes fun.

COURAGE

It takes courage to step forward. Having the courage and setting the intention for change is like putting a flag in the ground and announcing, "I'm here. Let me begin."

Your health journey is a story that unfolds day by day. Each choice, each decision, matters. In order to move forward, take the time to sincerely ask yourself, "What obstacles are in my way? What old stories, excuses, bad habits, and outdated ways of eating are standing between the me of today and the me I want to be?"

Now breathe, get quiet, listen to your inner voice. Trust that voice, be compassionate to it, that YOU, and ask yourself, "What is the one step I can take to move forward to regain my health and live a more vibrant life?"

Start with something simple, something concrete. You can choose to go through your pantry and throw out all the processed, sugar-laden, chemical-infused foods that are causing you to feel sick and be fat. Maybe you choose to call a trusted friend and ask them to be your support buddy. Or maybe you simply read the next chapter in this book to learn a bit about basic nutrition and enjoy the process of opening your mind to a whole new way of thinking.

What I know for sure from the success my clients achieve is that courage takes stepping out of your fear, out of your old habits, out of your outdated thoughts, out of your comfort zone, and into trust. That's where the magic happens.

MY BIG, MESSY LIFE MOMENT

For me, 2018 was a year of love, loss, pain, sorrow, friendship, expansion, and change. Moving out into my own place after a twenty-year marriage was a huge leap of faith into the unknown. It led me forward into new territory, new landscapes, new relationships, and to new opportunities that opened me up in places I didn't even know were closed. It was scary and exciting at the same time.

The decision to move into my own place was not an easy one. I remember wondering whether to sign the lease, so I called my friend Martin, who listened attentively to me then replied, "You need to *breathe*. Take some time for you. Give yourself some space."

And that's what I did.

After experiencing my breast cancer journey, a marriage that was extremely challenged, and the loss of my mother in October of 2017 (which came three months after her stage IV ovarian cancer diagnosis) I decided YES, I indeed needed the space to grieve, breathe, and reconnect with ME— from a place of love, from a place of self-care, from a place of remembering who I am, what lights me up, what my special gifts are, and how best to use them.

With each passing month, I met new people, had new experiences, traveled more, dove deeper into my business, got bolder in my conversations, hired a coach, went to therapy, and stepped through "walls of fire" that were unbelievably uncomfortable, scary, and anxiety-provoking—like the autumn evening I stood on stage at a breast cancer fundraiser and introduced my surgeon, Dr. Kristi Funk, as the guest speaker to an audience of 150 women. Many of those women were or are clients, colleagues, and friends. With Dr. Funk by my side, I shared the story of my breast cancer journey in public for the first time.

At the same time, those moments took me to new heights, new levels of confidence (like finding my voice and no longer holding myself back or worrying about what others would think), and realigned me with my truth—

ultimately allowing me to take off the armor surrounding my heart that I had been wearing for so long.

Being on my own for the first time in a small, cozy, charming, comfortable, safe, nurturing place allowed me to open my eyes to the beauty inside me and in others. Things became clearer that year. I began to see with wholehearted conviction that we are all connected; that we all crave love, affection, and validation; that we all come from families that have secrets, trauma, dysfunction, and pain; and that we all have unmet needs. Sometimes these things are talked about in the open, and sometimes they are hidden away in a box, in a secret letter, in a painful place of the heart, or in a hard-to-reach corner of the soul.

Creating change that year was one of the greatest gifts I ever gave to myself.

FINDING THE COURAGE WITHIN

LESLIE: AGE FIFTY, MOM, FITNESS TRAINER, ATLANTA, GEORGIA

"A new lease on life!"

When Leslie first called me, she felt sluggish, anxious, bloated, toxic, overweight, and completely out of balance. She also had a lot of sugar cravings and was longing to find more passion in her day-to-day experience of life. Leslie filled her day with chips, cookies, an abundance of pasta, and processed protein bars.

To begin, I put Leslie on my 21-day transformational food cleanse, taught her how to eat better, and inspired her to let go of excess sugar and chemicals by making healthier choices that nourished her body and satisfied her cravings. I also spent time teaching Leslie about the power of using breath as a tool to reduce stress and calm down her nervous system. I asked her to pause throughout the day to take breath breaks.

The breath breaks would consist of stopping, pausing, taking a deep, glorious, "fill up the lungs" breath, holding it for a second or two, and slowly releasing it. Then repeat two more times.

Sounds simple—but it made a powerful impact on Leslie's life. Deep breathing combined with a healthier way of eating opened up a new world for Leslie, and she began to feel better than she had in years.

During our coaching journey, Leslie released unwanted weight, increased her energy, reduced her sugar cravings, balanced her moods, and most of all created way more joy in her life. She also began to experience more inner peace and approached life from a new positive perspective.

One morning during our coaching conversation Leslie shared this: "Marlyn, with my new way of eating and living, I'm feeling calm, fit, and happy. What I'm noticing most is I have lost my sugar cravings, am making much healthier food choices, and when I'm going about my day I feel joyful for no special reason. I'm my happiest, too, when I'm working out."

Since Leslie expressed that she loved to exercise and was ready to take on a new career, I encouraged her to step outside her comfort zone and get trained as a certified fitness trainer— which she did! Now, in addition to maintaining her own nourishing lifestyle plan, she loves sharing her simple solutions and healthy lifestyle tools with her friends and clients. Leslie dug deep, found her courage, and stuck with it. And as a result, she gained incredible confidence, became more joyful, and created a new lease on life.

This is a big one: **Courage.** Because courage also takes letting go of self-criticism, releasing shame, and carving out the time for YOU.

"HOW DO I DO THAT?" YOU ASK.

One day at a time. One meal at a time. One decision at a time. One kind word to yourself at a time. (I am love. I am enough. I am worthy. I deserve health and well-being.)

GIVE YOURSELF PERMISSION.

You don't need to worry about what other people are thinking, and you don't need their permission to act on what you know to be true and necessary. All you need to do is give yourself permission to stop, slow down, and create some space. Day by day you'll become clear about what's important in your precious life. You can begin to set intentions and boundaries. You can give yourself permission to take that next step.

JUST SAY NO

One of the best tips I can offer you on your journey to better health is to have the courage to say no. No can be a very difficult word for many of us—maybe for all of us at one time or another. But cultivating the ability to say no at the appropriate times is a crucial step in taking ownership of our lives.

We learn how to say no by getting quiet, slowing down our breath, and tuning into our bodies and our minds.

When no is the response calling your heart, you say it, do it, live it, breathe it, even if it's uncomfortable. You will build your no muscle over time, just like you build a muscle at the gym by repeatedly lifting weights. It's the same thing here.

Your ability to get clear, get stronger, listen to your intuition, and say no when it's called for is built upon repetition over time. From that place you build strength and more confidence.

WHEN TEMPTATIONS APPEAR

Have you ever struggled with saying no to all the temptations that suddenly appear when you are changing your diet? What caused you to cave? How did you feel afterward?

The inability to say no is where I watch many people fall down the rabbit hole.

You want to say no to that plate of fries, rich creamy pasta dish, sugar-infused dessert, and that tall glass of Chardonnay, but you end up saying yes, and before you know it, you're saying, "Well, I might as well finish this bread basket, or fill in the blank, and start again on Monday."

Sound familiar?

HOW ABOUT FOMO?

HAVE YOU EVER STRUGGLED WITH THE FEAR OF MISSING OUT?

You're out with your friends and they're digging into that basket of crusty Italian bread, dipping slices into a bowl of olive oil with abandon. So far so good. You're thoughtfully ignoring it all until they order that second glass of wine for you. Or maybe you're at a party with fabulous hors d'oeuvres and you're tempted, caught up in the moment, piling your plate high with savory puff pastry treats. Before you know it, you've thrown your plan out the window, and you're right there digging into it all. After all, you'll start again on Monday.

FOMO can be a big problem for some if we're unaware of its hold.

The key to conquering FOMO is to know we have a choice. To be clear in our decisions and to know that the cocktail, bread basket, and gooey piece of chocolate cake will be there for you another time, if you so choose. That your true friends will love you no matter what (and may even be inspired by your actions). That your decision to be true to *you* first is more important than *any* temptation or worries we all have about what other people will think.

Success builds on success. Science has debunked that cliché. Each time you overcome these obstacles, your brain releases a shot of serotonin, the feel-good hormone. As you become happier with your accomplishments, you'll naturally build more self-confidence and pride.

Tap into that power, and you will have renewed energy to reach your larger goals. There is no downside. And whatever path you've chosen, there's a very good chance that you'll be happier and feel healthier than you've felt in years.

RADIANT TIP

NOTICE THE POSITIVE

When you find yourself taking any positive action steps, especially ones that are out of your norm, stop, pause, and notice. Notice any good feelings coming up—feelings of accomplishment, a job well-done, or a sense of pride. That noticing is how we start to build better habits. Because let's face it, we humans love to be noticed and validated for our positive traits. Why not celebrate them, big and small, and give yourself a pat on the back while you're at it? You are beautiful.

DIANA'S WELLNESS STORY: "PROJECT FIFTY AND FABULOUS."

On a beautiful autumn day in September 2019, Diana sat across from me on a comfy, brushed-velvet green chair in my home office. Warm sunlight beamed through the window and brightened up the room. I listened deeply as Diana shared how she was ready to make some serious changes with her food, health, and lifestyle. What she really desired more than anything was to lose twenty pounds and feel joy. Somewhere along the way of her busy life, raising kids, and having a full-time teaching and law career, she had gained weight and lost her joy.

Diana had been to many of my Project Radiance wellness events and even worked with me for a short while in 2010. This time was different. She was about to turn fifty. In fact, she named her wellness journey Project Fifty and Fabulous.

As I began to coach Diana, we looked at all areas of her life, including her work, marriage, motherhood role, and, most importantly, her relationship with herself. We concluded there was lots of room for positive change, especially in the area of self-care.

Join Diana and me in the pages ahead as we follow her journey of transformation.

Starting Off: I put Diana on my 21-day transformational food cleanse and cleaned up her high-carb diet. Our goal was to help her shed the excess weight and support her in feeling more energized each day. I also gave her the assignment of infusing "me time" into her calendar, as she was neglecting to make the space for herself. Beyond that, her life was filled with many demands and high-stress activities such as raising two teenage girls, running a family law practice, and being the CEO of her household.

As a way to get her connected to her wellness journey on a deeper level, I asked Diana what she was ready to release from her life, and she shared the following:

"I'm ready to release negativity and regrets about the past, disappointment with myself and others, and DIET MENTALITY. And the last is a big one, because I grew up in a household with a mother where diet mentality was prominent. My mom was either on a diet, or off her diet. There was no in between. That seems to be how I've been living my life as well. On or off. Black or white. No gray zone."

When I asked Diana about her goals, she said, "I want to become a mediator, develop a consistent commitment to positive change, and be open and willing to totally change the life I've been living. I also want to unapologetically love my life, create more joy and happiness, develop fit, toned arms, and eat for pleasure and health instead of boredom and stress."

And last, I asked Diana to take a moment to get clear about her *why* and write down the core reasons she was doing this wellness journey in the first place. If there was ever a point along the way where she wanted to throw in the towel, she could review the reasons she said yes to herself, and stay on track.

Her response...

My "WHY": Have fun, feel vibrant, lower inflammation, feel calm, energized, and rested, feel fit and strong, have "eating clean" be an integrated part of my life—it's just who I am in the world. I also want to look sensational, feel incredible, enjoy the journey and avoid looking at it as a destination, and, lastly, be unapologetically happy!"

Things started out great with Diana, and then we ran into a few challenges. We'll revisit Diana's journey in Chapter 4.

COMMITMENT

Perhaps the greatest struggle my clients run up against on their road to better health, wellness, and weight loss is staying committed.

Have you struggled with commitment as well?

You've taken that first step and have been following your new routine. You're leaving the honeymoon stage. You really want to change, but you're having trouble staying committed to your goals, integrating new habits into your life, and sustaining them over time. It's during the commitment phase where failure most often happens.

Why is it so difficult to stay committed? What causes us to veer off track? How do we let go and stop being so hard on ourselves when we've slipped? And what does it take to be *in it* for the long haul?

From my experience, staying committed to our dietary goals and ourselves means setting strong intentions and boundaries, making good choices day in and day out, letting go of the idea of perfection, having compassion for ourselves, and being aware of self-sabotage, food triggers, situation triggers, and people triggers. Most of all, it means supporting *your* individual body's nutritional and cellular needs, and no giving up—no matter what.

HOW TO STAY COMMITTED

1. Set strong boundaries and intentions.
2. Make good choices daily.
3. Let go of perfection and aim to do your best each day.
4. Have compassion for yourself. You are human.
5. Be aware of self-sabotage (food triggers, situation triggers, people triggers).
6. Support YOUR body's nutritional needs.
7. NO GIVING UP—no matter what! Adopt a stick-to-itiveness attitude.
8. If you break your rules, start again.

The only way you fail is if you quit.

DEBBIE: AGE FORTY-EIGHT, EXECUTIVE BANKER, LOS ANGELES, CALIFORNIA

"Discovering a healthier way to eat and live!"

Debbie was referred to me by a former client. When Debbie and I first met, she was tired, had severe back pain, and carried extra weight, especially around the belly. She was making poor food choices throughout the day and eating too much sugar, especially around 4 p.m. and before bed when she would have her milk and cookies, a habit she had carried with her since grade school.

As I do with most of my clients, I put Debbie on my 21-day transformational food cleanse and introduced her to healthier blood sugar balancing afternoon snacks (see Chapter 9) and swapped out her milk and cookies for herbal tea and cinnamon gluten-free crackers—all while keeping her satisfied, fueled, and happy.

Once Debbie made the mental commitment to her own wellness and self-care, her life began to shift. Her confidence improved, her body began regaining hormonal balance, and her skin glowed like it had in her twenties.

After three months of working together, Debbie lost fifteen pounds, increased her energy, and no longer experienced the horrific chronic back pain that was interfering with her life.

During our last session, Debbie shared this: "It's been a remarkable journey in which I learned so much (as did my husband too!). It's truly unbelievable how much better my body and back feels and I'm thrilled for all the great changes. Thank you, Marlyn, for showing me a new and healthier way to eat and live."

SET YOURSELF UP FOR SUCCESS

Here is one of the key insights I've consistently found to be true: When we set ourselves up for success and make a long-term commitment, we must become keenly aware of who we are spending our time with.

As humans, we are tribal beings and thrive in community. Shaping our environment by surrounding ourselves with friends, family, and coworkers who have a positive mindset and value fitness, health, and wellness can be extremely influential on our path to better health.

Jim Rohn, renowned motivational speaker, suggests that we are the average of the five people we spend the most time with. Take a moment to stop and think about the five people with whom you spend the most time. Do they have a positive, healthy mindset? Are they eating well, living well, and taking care of their body, mind, and spirit? Whose lifestyle habits do you admire the most? Why? Get curious. This is a great exercise to help us see how our outer world is a reflection of our inner world, and vice versa. Commitment to a new path becomes easier when we have the tools.

ILENE: AGE FIFTY-FIVE, HEALTHCARE SPECIALIST, MOM, BALTIMORE, MARYLAND

"It's never too late to change your health!"

When Ilene first called me, she felt pretty awful. Her weight was up, her blood sugar was off, her liver enzymes were skyrocketing, and her blood pressure was elevated. She also experienced a lot of heartburn. Because her diet regimens were just not working, her doctor suggested she get a nutritionist to help her learn new ways of eating and living.

Ilene decided to work with me and step into a more empowered approach to health. To start, I put Ilene on my 21-day standard protocol and within one week she began to feel better. After four months, Ilene lost thirty-five pounds, went from a size 12 to a size 6, and had a lot more energy for all the things she loved, including her husband and two beautiful daughters. On top of that, she began sleeping better, feeling happier, and upping her self-care by exercising more and choosing better snacks and meals while traveling for work.

To help her gain control and stay on track, I shared ways to incorporate her favorite foods and pleasurable desserts using the Three-Bite Rule (see Chapter 11) and suggested she give herself permission to have little cheats now and then, like her favorite sweet potato fries and a few bites of dessert as desired.

Within six months, Ilene's liver enzymes returned to normal, her blood sugar was lowered to optimal ranges, and her blood pressure was down—and no more heartburn either. With her old diet plans, the blood numbers never changed because those plans didn't focus on her body's needs. It was simply about losing weight and never focused on health at the deeper level.

In the pages to come, I'll share more about healthy blood sugar metabolism, insulin resistance, estrogen detoxification, and intermittent fasting. I'll explain what they are, why you need to be aware of them, and how they are all connected to your weight, energy, health, and emotional well-being.

Change happens when you have a system, a clear route, and someone to guide you. It's exciting. It's possible. It's doable.

Are you ready to courageously take that next step forward? Let's get educated on how the body works. I've got my favorite whiteboard and big beautiful easel with colorful erasable markers (blue, purple, orange, red, green) all set up for you.

Chapter 3

THE AGING METABOLISM

*"Take care of your body.
It's the only place you have to live."*

- JIM ROHM

What causes aging?

Why do some people age faster than others?

What has us gaining weight, getting sick, and feeling tired?

And how can we slow down and even reverse aging?

Let me take you behind the scenes and shine a light on how the body works on a cellular level.

In the spirit of keeping it simple, we'll join in on a fun adventure—*a journey*—where I'll share the most important things to know and the action steps to take to help you age well and feel your best. By having a clear picture of the science and systems that run our metabolic processes, we become empowered with the knowledge to make better choices as we move through midlife and beyond.

AGING WELL AND STRONG ...
AND WITH RADIANCE

WHAT IS RADIANCE?

Radiance is a glow, from either a light source like the sun or a healthy, beaming person. Radiance is an attractive combination of good health and happiness.

The quality of being bright and sending out rays of light from every cell in our bodies.

Aging strong and with stellar health starts on the inside and expresses itself on the outside, like the golden light of the sun.

Instead of a Band-Aid approach to fixing a problem, we want to get to the root cause. We're going to ask ourselves, what are the causes of high cholesterol, high blood pressure, and high blood sugar? We're going to ask if we truly need the medications prescribed to alleviate the symptoms. And if we do need them, we'll ask how we can better balance our diets and lifestyles to lead to healing.

Most importantly, we're going to find out why imbalances are happening. And we're going to learn simple strategies to heal. Perhaps that means shifting the foods we're eating, upgrading our lifestyle habits, cutting out sugar, getting more sleep, or moving our bodies.

POWER IN OUR HANDS

By understanding the simple concepts that run the body and rule the aging process, we have a better chance of taking positive steps and making better decisions for our long-term health and wellness.

As long as we are alive, we're going to age. Period. If we want to age well, we've got to embrace aging. And we had better do it with good health. Because investing in good health now will pay off in dividends for years to come.

KEY COMPONENTS OF AGING,
OR THE THINGS THAT CAUSE US TO AGE

- Oxidative stress/inflammation
- Hormonal imbalance
- Stress hormones
- Glucose/insulin regulation

- Immune balance
- Toxins/environmental burden
- Individuality

RADIANT TIP

UNDERSTAND THE ROOT CAUSE

Take the time to understand the root cause of your symptoms, and learn to understand any medications and pills you've been prescribed. True healing begins when you understand and address your symptoms, and create the right diet, exercise plan, and mental outlook.

OPTIMAL MIDLIFE AGING:METABOLISM ROADMAP
EVERYTHING IS CONNECTED!

When one area or system of the body doesn't work properly, it can have a major effect on other areas. Think of the body as an interconnected highway system. When roads are open and traffic is light, cars, trucks, and buses flow freely. When accidents happen or roads are blocked, traffic may slow down, get backed up, or even get diverted to other roads. This can have a major effect on how things flow for the day or over time. Like those roadways, we want the pathways in our bodies to flow freely in their daily activities (such as metabolism, digestion, elimination) and remain free from blockages and disruptions.

STEP 1: UNDERSTANDING METABOLISM
AND HOW IT WORKS

WHAT IS METABOLISM, ANYWAY?
METABOLISM 101

Your metabolism takes the food you eat (nutrients) and the oxygen you breathe and turns them into energy. In other words, metabolism is the process where food is digested by, assimilated by, and eliminated from the body. Your metabolism keeps you alive, nourished, heated, and full of energy. And as we age, our metabolic system (metabolism) begins to slow down.

SIGNS AND SYMPTOMS OF AN AGING METABOLISM

These may include:
- weight gain
- insulin resistance (weakened response to insulin and glucose)
- metabolic syndrome (cardiovascular risk factors)
- poor digestion
- poor sleep
- lack of focus
- lack of energy

A few of these symptoms are considered a "normal" part of aging. And here's the GOOD NEWS: most of these areas are mu*ch more under our control* than we've been taught.

Women need to remember that we may need to care for ourselves differently than we did when we were twenty or thirty, especially if we want to preserve our energy, beauty, and overall good health. More priority must be given to how we eat and nourish our changing bodies.

We've got to give more to get more. Think about it. Do you want a vibrant sex life, high energy to do the things you love, and a body that carries you forward into old age? If the answer is yes, that means bringing more conscious choices into your everyday life.

Our body is a beautiful piece of machinery, accomplishing amazing tasks day in and day out. Over time as we grow older, our bodies slow down and may need tending to in new ways. Some parts may even need to be upgraded or replaced (like a knee or hip replacement). We want our bodies to run *well* over the course of our lives. This might mean doing things differently than we have in years past. This might mean being kinder, eating different foods or less carbs, adding in more plants, taking a few new supplements, or scheduling more time for rest and healing. We want to keep our machinery well-oiled and running smoothly now and into our later years.

A MAP OF OUR CELLS AND HOW THEY WORK

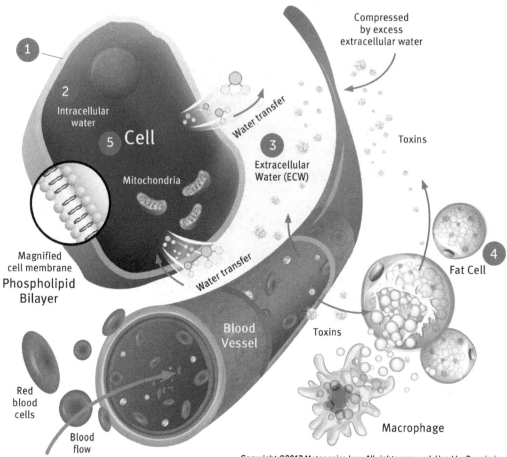

1. **Phase Angle:** The outer rim of the cell. A healthy phase angle is pliable and allows things to move in and out of the cell easily. Fish oil (from fish and quality supplements) supports a healthy phase angle.
2. **Intracellular Water:** The water/hydration inside the cell.
3. **Extracellular Water:** The water/hydration outside the cell. (We want good/easy water transfer in and out.)
4. **Fat Cell:** Houses toxins. (Think of your fat cells as a storage unit. We want to avoid high amounts of fat and high amounts of toxins being stored.)
5. **Muscle Cell:** Muscle cells are where our active metabolism is happening throughout the body. Our job is to get them functioning well.

RADIANT TIP

Your actions CAN make a difference in how you age

What you eat and how you live can slow down the aging process. And that is very good news.

STEP 2: UNDERSTANDING ENERGY AND MITOCHONDRIA

Where does our energy come from and how can we create more?

MITOCHONDRIA 101

Mitochondria are the powerhouse energy-makers of the cell. As we age, we need to make sure our cells and mitochondria are functioning well. This is a vital component of supporting and maintaining our optimal energy and health.

Mitochondria are tiny cell structures (sub-compartments called organelles within the cell) that take the food we eat and the oxygen we breathe, break them down, digest them, and turn them into energy. Think of mitochondria as the digestive system within the cell. Mitochondria exist within each cell (see chart above) and in active organs like muscles, heart, and the brain. The mitochondria make your metabolism happen.

Mitochondria are VITAL to health. You need energy to do all the things you love each day—to breathe, sleep, eat, play, and lose weight. If your mitochondria are not working properly, your body will produce less energy, or none at all. When there is no energy, there is no life.

As we age, the mitochondria begin to break down and their function within the cell declines.

The good thing to know is that we can do something about this. We can protect our cells and our mitochondria from breaking down quickly and aging too fast.

HOW DO WE PROTECT OUR MITOCHONDRIA AS WE AGE?

There are three primary strategies to optimize mitochondrial function and maintain or improve energy production.

1. **Reduce exposure to damaging factors** such as heavy metals (lead, mercury, cadmium), organic pollutants (paint fumes, detergents, new carpet fumes), and cigarette smoke.

2. **Provide the necessary nutrition** to support mitochondria function.

3. **Provide protection from oxidative damage** by supporting the body with antioxidants.

WHAT ARE ANTIOXIDANTS AND WHY SHOULD WE CARE?

Antioxidants are compounds that help prevent or slow down damage to our cells caused by free radicals. Free radicals are waste substances produced by cells. When free radicals float through our system unchecked, they can wreak havoc on our health and cause oxidative stress, sometimes leading to disease, illness, and/or cancer. Antioxidants help neutralize and stabilize those free radicals, thus preventing them from causing damage.

- **Antioxidants help heal, repair, and support strong mitochondria.** They also support longevity and help us age well. Our bodies are designed to make their own antioxidants including glutathione and alpha-lipoic acid. The foods we eat supply other antioxidants, like vitamin E and vitamin C.

- **Antioxidants are found in colorful plants, vegetables, herbs, spices, and fruits like berries and citrus.** Antioxidants are also found in coffee, green tea, and dark chocolate (YAY!). We want to fill our plates with high amounts of antioxidants. A plant-rich diet is an excellent way to take in more antioxidants. (Note: You can still eat animal protein. We just want to focus on high amounts of plants for health and healing.)

RADIANT TIP

GET SOME GLUTATHIONE

Glutathione (aka, the mother of all antioxidants) is one of the body's most important antioxidants, because it helps to maintain our intracellular health. Glutathione is present in every cell of our body and helps play a key role in inflammation and immunity. Although glutathione is produced by the body, it can get depleted as we age. Many things can deplete glutathione levels, including poor diet, stress, and ongoing infections. Below are a few ways to support and increase healthy glutathione levels naturally.

1. Eat sulfur-rich foods like steak, fish, broccoli, cauliflower, and garlic.
2. Up your vitamin C intake with vitamin C supplements.
3. Add in selenium-rich foods, like Brazil nuts and brown rice.
4. Consume foods naturally rich in glutathione, like spinach, avocados, and asparagus.
5. Consider adding in a liposomal glutathione supplement. (The liposomal delivery system protects the glutathione from breaking down in the digestive tract.)

RADIANT TIP

MIND YOUR MITOCHONDRIA

Love your mitochondria. For better energy and a higher functioning metabolism, eat more antioxidant-rich foods like blueberries, cacao, kiwi, papaya, parsley, oolong tea, and matcha green tea. Support your mitochondria with restorative sleep and a healthy lifestyle. Include supplements, if needed. Your mitochondria will be happy and thank you.

RADIANT TIP

HEALTHY FAT, FUEL FOR MITOCHONDRIA

Healthy fats like avocados, olive oil, flaxseed oil, and oily fish like wild salmon protect the mitochondria and fuel the brain by providing anti-inflammatory support.

Note: For some, mitochondria supplementation may be necessary and/or helpful.

Not everyone needs to take supplements. If your energy is low, the following supplements can support better mitochondria. (See Chapter 8 for more information on supplements.)

VITAMINS AND MINERALS
FOR HEALTHY MITOCHONDRIA AND ENERGY

- Vitamin B complex
- Magnesium
- Glutathione
- Alpha-lipoic acid
- Coenzyme Q10

- D-ribose
- Phosphatidylcholine
- NAD (nicotinamide adenine dinucleotide)

STEP 3: UNDERSTANDING BLOOD SUGAR, INSULIN, AND INFLAMMATION

How does metabolism change as we age?

BLOOD SUGAR METABOLISM 101

As we hit midlife, our bodies change. Women generally have a harder time metabolizing the sugars from the food and alcohol we consume. Declining hormones and overconsumption of sugar and carbohydrates through the years leads to a weakened response to insulin. This can then lead to health problems, including diabetes, pre-diabetes, high blood pressure, weight gain, high cholesterol, and unbalanced hormones.

WHAT IS BLOOD SUGAR?

Our bodies use blood sugar, also known as glucose, to create energy within our cells.

WHAT IS INSULIN?

Insulin is a hormone produced in the pancreas. It lowers blood sugar by driving glucose and other nutrients into cells, especially muscle cells. Your muscles need glucose to help them produce energy and recover from the effects of exercise. Think of insulin as the key that unlocks the cell membrane door. The response of the cell to insulin is *critically* important to blood sugar metabolism.

HEALTHY BLOOD SUGAR METABOLISM

Achieving and maintaining proper blood sugar metabolism is essential for a lifetime of excellent health. With normal, healthy digestion, unrefined carbohydrates (carbohydrates in their whole with fiber attached) are broken down to smaller sugars and are then absorbed through the intestines into the blood. This stimulates the pancreas to secrete an appropriate amount of insulin into the blood, which facilitates the delivery of sugar into the cells throughout the body.

When insulin binds to insulin receptors that are attached to the cell membrane, a signal is sent to sugar transport systems inside the cell. The sugar transport channels allow for effective sugar delivery from the blood into the cell. The sugar then enters the cell and is used for energy production by the mitochondria or is stored for further use.

UNHEALTHY BLOOD SUGAR METABOLISM

When we eat refined carbohydrates (carbohydrates that have been processed and stripped of their natural fiber), they are broken down and absorbed very quickly and can cause a rapid increase in our blood sugar. When blood sugar is high, the pancreas responds by producing additional insulin in an effort to help sugar get into the cell and do its job. In unhealthy blood sugar metabolism, the cell may be unresponsive to the insulin. The pancreas then tries to produce even more insulin. Over time, continual high levels of insulin can lead to increased triglyceride levels, decreased HDL ("good") cholesterol levels, and hormone imbalances.

Faulty sugar metabolism can affect the health of our eyes, nerves, blood vessels, kidneys, and pancreas. It can also impact our weight, body shape, energy levels, blood pressure, cholesterol, triglycerides, and cardiovascular health.

Factors that contribute to unhealthy blood sugar metabolism:

1. Obesity
2. Lack of exercise
3. Unhealthy diet with too many refined sugars and fast-burning carbs

Note: Many of us find that as we get older, those baskets of fried chips and bread we once enjoyed with our glass of Chardonnay no longer sit well in our guts. It may be time to check our insulin levels. All of which is to say, enjoy your treats, but be aware of how many refined and high-glycemic carbohydrates you're consuming (fast burning, quickly digested and absorbed carbs, like candy and chips). When choosing foods, consider options containing lower carbohydrates (slow-burning, slowly digested and absorbed carbs, like berries and sweet potatoes).

INSULIN RESISTANCE 101 (IMPORTANT TO KNOW!)

WHAT IS INSULIN RESISTANCE?

Insulin resistance means that your cells are not fully responsive to insulin when it signals them to let in glucose (blood sugar). Recall that insulin is the key that unlocks the cell wall to allow glucose to do its work. With insulin resistance, the key can't effectively unlock the cells. As a result, your blood sugar starts to rise. Your pancreas responds by releasing more insulin. When insulin resistance outpaces the ability of your pancreas to produce more insulin, diabetes occurs.

Whether or not you actually develop diabetes, high levels of circulating insulin can have seriously negative effects. High insulin levels make the kidneys retain fluid, raise blood pressure, and create that feeling of being bloated and swollen. High insulin levels prevent cells from breaking down fat, making it harder to lose weight through dieting. With insulin resistance, some sugar gets into the cell, some goes to the liver, and some gets stored as fat.

WHAT CAUSES INSULIN RESISTANCE?

After we turn forty, our bodies may respond less and less to insulin because we have less muscle in which to burn glucose. For some of us who have a challenging time losing weight, this is also known as weight loss resistance.

When we develop insulin resistance, the cells in our muscles don't receive enough blood sugar to function properly. They no longer efficiently burn the sugar that circulates in our blood. Insulin also turns on genes that produce molecules that control the generation, maintenance, and resolution of inflammation. With high insulin, the level of inflammation in our body increases.

Inflammation occurs when we are under stress. Inflammation disrupts the body's harmony. Inflammation interferes with the effect of insulin on our muscles.

Our brain and adrenal glands are attuned to the level of inflammation in our body. As inflammation increases, our brain sends a signal to our adrenal glands to produce more of a hormone called cortisol. You may be familiar with cortisone, a drug used to relieve symptoms of inflammation like itching, redness, or pain. Cortisol is the natural equivalent of the drug, made in our own adrenal glands in response to stress. Cortisol combats inflammation, but at a high price. **Cortisol increases the amount of belly fat.** It also causes fluid retention, muscle weakness, memory loss, high blood pressure, and further raises your blood sugar. The increase in blood sugar then stimulates a further increase in insulin. If consistently unattended to, this becomes a vicious cycle.

INSULIN RESISTANCE + SEX HORMONES

Sugar raises insulin levels and creates a hormonal domino effect that knocks our sex hormones—estrogen, progesterone, and testosterone—out of balance. Sex hormones, healthy blood sugar, and insulin balance are all connected. Spikes in insulin and the insulin resistance that results from eating too much sugar and refined flour can lead to unwanted issues like acne, irregular menstrual cycles, weight gain, fatigue, and hair loss. Rebalancing these hormones is possible when we change what we put on our plates.

RADIANT TIP

INSULIN + BLOOD TESTS

If you don't know your fasting insulin level, request a blood test to find out.

Make insulin your friend. Be aware of carbs.

Be careful, too, with the good carbs. Modify intake. Move your body.

A PERSONAL STORY

One of the hardest lessons for me was realizing that I can no longer eat carbs in the same way I could when I was younger. Even too much of the good stuff, like brown rice, whole fruit, or sweet potatoes, will raise my blood sugar. In my twenties and thirties, I was able to go to a Chinese restaurant and have a great big serving (or two) of delicious vegetable fried rice. Now my body responds differently. My rice portion must stay around 1/2 cup to keep my blood sugar balanced. I've also switched from fried rice to steamed brown rice. The lesson is simple: If we continue into midlife with our same high-carb food habits, we will flood our body with too much sugar (glucose)!

Of course, once in a while, the pleasure of a beautiful meal or decadent dessert is worth every calorie and carb, like when I return home to Philly for Thanksgiving and have some of my Aunt Ilene's amazing homemade apple pie. But if we live from a place of overindulgence day in and day out, we will pay the price.

If you are struggling with weight loss, it's worth your while to look at your carbs. How many are you eating a day?

RADIANT TIP

FIND YOUR TIPPING POINT

There is no perfect level of carb consumption. Here is one area where metabolism is different for each and every one of us. On the days I work out with weights or do more extensive exercise like a long hike, my body craves more complex carbohydrates such as quinoa, sweet potatoes, or brown rice. On other days, I might need less. Remember that part of your radiant journey is to *find your tipping point*, the place where *you and your body* thrive.

Picture Goldilocks and her bowl of porridge. You're aiming for not too much, not too little, but just the right amount. Sometimes that might look like three to four bites of a carb-rich food like Aunt Sarah's ninetieth birthday carrot cake with cream cheese frosting. Sometimes it may be a small sweet potato, perhaps with a bit of sweet cream butter or some coconut butter. Or maybe it's a bit more quinoa on exercise days and none on other days.

Bottom line: We want to find the place where we feel good and energized and our weight and blood sugar stays stable.

RADIANT TIP

4 KEY AREAS THAT AFFECT A WOMAN'S METABOLISM AS SHE AGES

1. Hormones
2. Loss of muscle
3. Lack of sleep
4. Insulin resistance

STEP 4: UNDERSTANDING METABOLIC SYNDROME

METABOLIC SYNDROME 101

WHAT IS METABOLIC SYNDROME?

Metabolic Syndrome is a cluster of cardiovascular risk factors that often occur when insulin resistance and obesity come into play.

What contributes to metabolic syndrome?

1. High-carb, high saturated fat diet
2. Physical inactivity (sedentary lifestyle)
3. Obesity
4. Genetic factors

SIGNS OF METABOLIC SYNDROME

Metabolic syndrome is present if you have three or more of the following signs:

1. Elevated blood pressure
2. Elevated blood glucose
3. Enlarged waist circumference (for women, 35 inches or more)
4. Low HDL (good) cholesterol (for women, under 50 mg/dl)
5. Elevated triglycerides (equal to or higher than 150 mg/dl)

What is the treatment for metabolic syndrome?

1. Diet
2. Exercise
3. Lifestyle
4. Weight loss
5. If you are a smoker, it's essential to stop smoking!

NOTE: Individuals who do not respond to lifestyle changes may need medication to treat metabolic syndrome, insulin resistance, high blood pressure, or high cholesterol.

STEP 5: UNDERSTANDING HORMONES AND THE BODY SYSTEMS THAT SUPPORT THEM

HORMONES 101: THE CHEMICAL MESSENGERS

We are made up of a complex symphony of hormones—estrogen, progesterone, testosterone, thyroid, and more. When these chemical messengers unite in harmony, we experience optimally functioning health. As we move into our perimenopausal and menopausal years, our hormones will begin to shift. This shift usually begins slowly in our thirties, with more dramatic changes happening in our forties, fifties, and sixties. Often accompanying these changes, we see an increase in weight gain and a slower, more sluggish metabolism.

WOMEN, WEIGHT, AND HORMONES

The key to bringing your body, weight, and hormones under control is to start now and move those goals forward one step at a time. Small action steps over time lead to new habits.

Years ago, I read a phenomenal book called *Growth Mindset* by Carol Dweck. In it, Dweck teaches us the difference between a *set mindset*, one that says, "I don't have self-discipline. I can't do this. I'm not good at change," and a *growth mindset*, one that says, "I can do this. I may not be good at this today, though I can learn, and I'll do it differently tomorrow."

Dweck shares that a growth mindset can be cultivated. Over time, if we put our intentions toward change, we can develop our talents, modify our temperaments, access our inner landscapes, and master new skills. A growth mindset says, "I may have eaten too much chocolate (or drank too much wine) today, but tomorrow I'm going to do better." "I'll go to the gym and stay hydrated." "I'll see what I need to do to go for a promotion at work."

There are seven hormones that can affect our weight:

- Leptin
- Estrogen*
- Insulin*
- Cortisol*
- Thyroid
- Growth Hormone
- Testosterone

*Note: Estrogen, insulin, and cortisol are fat-storage hormones.

LEPTIN 101: THE FEEL FULL HORMONE

Leptin is the satiety hormone. It signals the brain to put down the fork and stop eating. For some of us, leptin stops working and the brain never gets the signal. The result is that we keep eating and never feel full. Often, this imbalance leads to a cycle where we keep eating the wrong foods in an addictive pattern and gain weight.

Enter our friend Insulin. Elevated insulin eventually leads to high leptin levels. So our first plan of action is to get our insulin levels in check. (**As you will continue to learn, most everything goes back to insulin, the leader of the hormone pack.**)

Aging also affects leptin, due to muscle mass decline. Muscle gets replaced by fat. Fat tells your brain to eat more food by making us less responsive to insulin and leptin signals. This is known as *leptin resistance*. Leptin resistance is now believed to be one of the major contributors to obesity.

HOW TO GET LEPTIN WORKING MORE EFFICIENTLY:

1. Have your insulin levels checked. Lower your carb intake.
2. Make time for exercise. Remember, your body was designed to move.
3. Aim for 7–8 hours of sleep. Less sleep = less leptin = hungrier you.
4. Avoid industrial oils like corn, soybean, and canola. These oils are linked to higher inflammation. They also have the potential to flip our metabolic switches and store fat. (I will share more in Chapter 5.)
5. Practice intermittent fasting, which helps regulate and reset certain hormones, especially insulin and leptin.
6. Lower your toxic load. Toxins/chemicals in our food, personal care products, and makeup can get stored in our fat cells. These disruptors are called obesogens. Obesogens affect leptin levels, making it a challenge to lose weight.

If you are having trouble losing weight or are experiencing hormones that are out of balance, the following supplements may help. Not everyone needs supplements. However, the right supplements targeted to support your specific hormonal imbalances can bring the body into balance.

How do we know what we need? Test, don't guess. In the next chapter we'll look at specific blood tests that will give us key information regarding hormones and health.

SUPPLEMENTS FOR BETTER BLOOD SUGAR REGULATION

- **Inositol:** 2 inositol tablets daily improves insulin sensitivity.
- **Myo-inositol:** 2 grams once or twice per day improves insulin sensitivity.

- **Vitamin D:** 2,000 or 5,000 IU per day depending on blood levels.
- **Chromium picolinate:** 200–1,000mg per day. Chromium acts as an insulin sensitizer and may help reverse insulin resistance.
- **Berberine:** A bioactive compound from plants, berberine activates an enzyme called AMP (activated protein kinase) inside our cells that plays a major role in regulating metabolism. For many, it causes a reduction in blood sugar levels and decreases insulin resistance. Berberine has a half-life, so it's recommended that you spread dosage throughout the day.
- **Omega 3:** Helps with blood sugar regulation and cellular health.

Note: If you have a medical condition or are on any medications, speak to your doctor before taking any of these supplements.

RADIANT TIP

FOR BETTER BALANCED BLOOD SUGAR

1. Eat a low-carb, low-glycemic diet.
2. Think protein, healthy fat, and fiber at meals and snack time.
3. Consider adding berberine, alpha-lipoic acid, and chromium to your diet.
4. Consider eating more fish, hemp seeds, or add in a supplement to ensure you get enough omega-3's

MY "AHA" MOMENT WITH FOOD AND FUNCTIONAL MEDICINE

In 2007, it was like the carnival lights coming on all at once when I first learned the principles of functional medicine and connected my blood sugar challenges and hormonal imbalances to how I lived, what I ate, and the supplements I needed to take to support my body. Everything was new and fresh. It was like going back to nutrition school. Nutrition was new and exciting again.

Food, nutrition, and health made so much more sense because **functional medicine looks at the whole person and how the systems in our bodies function** in concert with one another. Functional medicine gives us meaningful ways and simple actionable lifestyle interventions for positive change.

WHAT IS ESTROGEN AND WHY SHOULD WE CARE?

ESTROGEN 101: THE "FEMALE" HORMONE

The hormone estrogen supports brain health, bone health, heart health, sex drive, and various other properties in our bodies. Estrogen gives women breasts and hips and keeps our joints lubricated. And while women have the bulk of estrogen, men have estrogen too, in much smaller amounts.

THE EFFECT OF LOWER ESTROGEN IN MENOPAUSE

"I feel like I'm aging. I'm not myself anymore. I'm depressed and irritable. My sleep is messed up. I'm feeling uncomfortable in my skin."

When our ovaries begin retiring from their baby-making years, we come into perimenopause. And finally, when our periods stop, we enter menopause.

Most women will spend a full third of our lives in menopause. And before that, we'll go through perimenopause, where our estrogen levels begin the process of falling. On average, estradiol (active form of estrogen) levels before menopause are 30-400 picograms per milliliter (pg/mL). After menopause, estradiol levels fall below 30 pg/mL.

With lower levels of our "good" estrogen, middle body fat may increase. So it's important to pay attention to what we eat and the products we use. (Note: For some, a bit of body fat around the middle may be okay, and even protective. We have to find the balance between our naturally changing bodies and good health plus incorporating a healthy diet. Also, at this time of life, you may be interested in trying bioidentical or replacement hormones. This is a great subject to discuss with your physician or gynecologist.)

Those of us who have been through menopause know the positive effects of this part of our lives. We no longer have to worry about getting pregnant. We won't experience hormone spikes and mood swings before and after ovulation or the bloating that comes just before our periods start.

ESTROGEN: THE GOOD, THE BAD, THE UGLY

Estrone (E1): The weakest form of estrogen; made in the ovaries. After menopause, this is the only estrogen the body continues to make in limited amounts.

Estradiol (E2): The most potent form of estrogen, made in the ovaries during the reproductive years.

Estriol (E3): A weak estrogen produced by the placenta during pregnancy.

Estetrol (E4): A weak estrogen only produced by the fetus during pregnancy

Other forms of estrogen include:

- **Synthetic estrogens:** They are produced for medical use such as birth control bills.
- **Phytoestrogens:** They are found in plants like soy, red clover, and flaxseed.
- **Xenoestrogens:** These are endocrine-disrupting pollutants from man-made products.

RADIANT TIP

WHAT EXACTLY ARE XENOESTROGENS?

The chemicals and ingredients we want to be especially mindful of avoiding are xenoestrogens, or "foreign" estrogens. These foreign estrogens mimic our own estrogen and are also known as hormone disruptors. Some xenoestrogens have even been found to be carcinogenic.

Where are xenoestrogens found?

They are found in makeup, shampoos, nail polish, cleaning supplies, fragrances, perfumes, chemically scented candles and air fresheners, canned goods, cash register receipts, sunscreens, deodorants, and toothpastes. The kinds of chemicals to look for are parabens, phthalates, and BPA. For further information, check out EWG.org.

ESTROGEN METABOLISM

Once they do their job, estrogens are metabolized—mostly in the liver and in a few other tissues in the body. During the metabolization phase, estrogens can choose from one of these three pathways:

- 2-OH-E1: This is the healthy, protective pathway.
- 4-OH-E1: This is unfavorable and is the most reactive and can bind to and damage DNA, causing cancer.
- 16-OH-E1: This is unfavorable and is strong estrogenic activity. Studies show that it may increase the risk of breast cancer.

Our goal is to keep our 2-OH-E1 pathway as the main one to maintain balance in the body.

HOW TO OPTIMIZE YOUR ESTROGEN DETOXIFICATION PATHWAYS

Learning how to optimize one's detoxification system during midlife and beyond is essential for losing weight and creating lifelong vibrant health.

Poor gastrointestinal health can inhibit excretion of unwanted estrogen from the body and promote its reabsorption back up into the body, which can be a danger. This form of estrogen is more problematic.

By supporting the liver and the gut, we can influence the health of our bodies and our metabolism.

Liver and Gut Support:

1. **EGCG** from green tea
2. **DIM:** This is a compound generated from cruciferous vegetables like broccoli, cauliflower, and cabbage. This category of vegetables contains indole-3-carbinol, which our bodies metabolize upon digestion into diindolylmethane, or DIM. DIM helps to remind damaged cells that they should self-destruct (called apoptosis) because sometimes cells forget to do this, which can lead to cancer and/or disease. It can be difficult to get the high amounts of DIM needed to support this process just from vegetables alone, so **taking a supplement may be helpful.** DIM has been shown to reduce estrogen-based cancers such as breast and cervical cancer by

helping the body maintain a better balance of good and bad estrogen. Men can benefit from DIM too. It helps to avoid too much testosterone being converted into estrogen. This is especially true when there is high belly fat.

3. **Milk thistle**
4. **Sprouted seeds**
5. **Ground Flaxseeds**

TO CLEAR OUT BAD ESTROGEN:

Eat a lot of vegetables each day. (Think a pound!) The fiber in vegetables helps excrete estrogen so it doesn't keep circulating in the body. Be mindful that when you add more fiber, you might see more bloating at first. Drink plenty of water and stay hydrated. Over time, your system should normalize.

RADIANT TIP

MATCHA IS MAGICAL

Matcha contains chlorophyll, which helps improve our liver function and in turn helps improve our body's ability to flush out toxins. Chlorophyll has been shown to help with the excretion of heavy metals, dioxins, and other persistent chemicals, like PCBs. Drinking matcha tea is one of the most delicious ways to boost the body's detox abilities, every single day.

Other benefits of matcha:

- **Cancer-Kicking: Matcha contains catechins,** a unique set of antioxidants that are potent cancer-fighters. According to the National Cancer Institute, green tea is one of the most powerful cancer-fighters.
- **Calm and Focused:** Matcha is rich in L-theanine, which supports feeling calm and focused. Matcha contains about five times the amount of L-theanine found in other green and black teas.
- **Fat Burning:** Matcha has been shown to increase thermogenesis, the body's rate of burning calories. One study showed that drinking matcha before exercise resulted in 25 percent more fat being burned.

Try my Matcha Latte recipe in Chapter 10.

PROGESTERONE 101: THE CALM HORMONE

Progesterone is a female sex hormone. Its primary function is to thicken the lining of the uterus each month to prepare the body for pregnancy. Progesterone also helps with metabolism, supports the thyroid, and gives us a nice sex drive. Think of progesterone as the calming, feel-good hormone. During perimenopause and menopause, progesterone levels decrease. Before menopause, our progesterone levels can range from .07/mL–25/mL, depending on what phase of the menstrual cycle we are in. After menopause, our levels drop to <.04/mL. When we are in menopause and our progesterone levels drop, we may experience more anxiety, increased bloat, sleepless nights, decreased sex drive, hot flashes, and weight gain. We may also feel more emotionally raw, vulnerable, and sensitive. Estrogen and progesterone are closely related. As our estrogen, progesterone, and testosterone levels change, so do we.

RADIANT TIP

HOW TO PROMOTE PROGESTERONE, NATURALLY

To support the body in making progesterone, maintain a healthy body weight and practice forms of stress reduction such as deep breathing, meditation, and yoga. Vitamin C and foods containing magnesium (dark chocolate, nuts, spinach) and vitamin B6 (broccoli, sweet potatoes, whole grains) are another way to promote the production of progesterone

TESTOSTERONE 101: THE FIERY SEX HORMONE

Testosterone is found predominantly in men, although women have testosterone too. It promotes muscles and bigger bones and supports our immune function. In women, testosterone is produced in the ovaries and adrenal glands. It's part of what makes us feel confident, strong, and sexy.

While women produce approximately 250 micrograms (0.25 milligrams) of testosterone a day, men usually produce ten to forty times that amount. But growing evidence supports that testosterone has a large role in our female desire. Think of testosterone as the heat that fires up our brains and makes us feel erotic and sensual.

Women often have more body fat than men. One function of our fat cells is to produce an enzyme called aromatase, which converts testosterone to estradiol. The more fat you have, the more likely you are to create an excess of androgens (testosterone) and estrogens. This is fine if your body is functioning normally. Some bodies however, my own included, have a tendency to convert testosterone into too much estrogen and that can lead to further problems (like estrogen-dependent breast cancer) if the estrogen is not properly eliminated from the body.

Here's where lifestyle choices come into play. When menopause hits, testosterone levels drop to half the levels they were before menopause. This is usually due to the decline in adrenal production. Even after the ovaries stop making certain forms of estrogen, they continue to make testosterone. As testosterone levels begin to dip, it is often accompanied by a higher sensitivity to stress, weight gain, changes in mood, and a lower libido. A few ways to raise your testosterone levels include lifting weights, getting plenty of restful deep quality sleep, minimizing stress and cortisol levels, and keeping vitamin D levels in the optimal range.

RADIANT TIP

WHITE BUTTON MUSHROOMS: THE POWERFUL AROMATASE INHIBITOR!

White button mushrooms are loaded with phytochemicals and isoflavones that help inhibit aromatase activity and breast cancer cell proliferation. A 2001 NIH study states that diets high in mushrooms (white button, shiitake, portobello, crimini, and baby mushrooms) may function in chemoprevention in postmenopausal women by reducing the in-cell production of estrogen.

Note: It is best to cook mushrooms.

MELATONIN 101: THE SLEEP HORMONE

Melatonin is an anti-aging hormone made by the pineal gland in the brain. It helps to maintain the body's circadian rhythm (sleep/wake cycle), regulates other hormones, and controls the timing and release of female reproductive hormones. Melatonin is synthesized from tryptophan, an essential amino acid. Melatonin has also been shown to seal the blood/brain barrier, the key barrier that keeps out toxins and other blood components that may disturb the brain. Melatonin has antioxidative activity and appears to be protective against a variety of cancers, including breast cancer.

How to raise melatonin levels:

1. Sleep in a dark room at night.
2. Limit screen time before bed. Turn off electronics at least one hour before bed. Blue light emitted from screens throws off our melatonin production.
3. Eat more melatonin-rich foods, like goji berries, walnuts, bananas, and dark cherries.
4. For some, it helps to take melatonin before bedtime. (Note: It's best to talk to your doctor about proper timing and dosing.)
5. Practice mindfulness techniques to keep your stress at bay and help keep your cortisol levels in check.

DHEA 101: THE VITALITY HORMONE

DHEA (dehydroepiandrosterone) is a hormone made by the body mainly in the adrenal glands but also in the ovaries (testes for men), skin, and brain. DHEA peaks in early adulthood (around age thirty) and then slowly falls over time as we age. DHEA can be made in a lab from chemicals found in wild yam and soy, though it cannot be manufactured by the body if we eat those foods. DHEA contributes to good skin health and higher energy levels. It has been studied to improve sexuality, vaginal health, menopause symptoms, well-being, metabolic syndrome, and weight loss. DHEA is still being tested, so as with any bioidentical hormone, speak with your doctor to see what is right for you.

CORTISOL 101: THE STRESS HORMONE

Cortisol is a steroid hormone produced in the adrenal glands and helps regulate stress. Cortisol also has a role in regulating metabolism, blood sugar levels, blood pressure, and immune response. Cortisol enables us to act quickly in times of stress, especially during fight or flight situations. But many of us lead stressful lives, and we often tend to produce too much cortisol.

Prolonged exposure to high levels of cortisol can have a direct effect on our weight, inflammation, and health. We tend to store fat when we have too much cortisol, especially in our bellies. High levels of cortisol can cause fluid retention, muscle weakness, memory loss, high blood pressure, and fatigue. In addition, high cortisol has been linked to depression, anxiety, food addiction, and sugar cravings.

Over time, high cortisol levels can lead to metabolic changes and insulin resistance. With chronically elevated cortisol, muscles don't respond to insulin in the same way. Instead of the muscles burning the fuel you've given them, they send it to the fat cells for safekeeping.

High cortisol has been shown to promote the aging process.

High cortisol breaks down muscles and ages us before our time.

SIGNS YOUR CORTISOL MAY BE ELEVATED:

1. You are unable to settle or relax.
2. You've noticed an increase in belly fat. You may even have developed a muffin top, that evocative term that paints a rather poetic picture of your belly spilling over your blue jeans.
3. Your cholesterol levels are higher than usual.
4. You're tired, but you can't sleep.
5. You are bloated and your body is retaining fluid.
6. You're experiencing lapses in memory.
7. Your blood sugar levels are higher than normal.

RADIANT TIP

TO LOWER CORTISOL

1. **Rest. Relax. Breathe.** This simple practice turns on the parasympathetic nervous system and helps the body get into a calmer place, which in turn helps to lower cortisol levels.
2. **Hit the pause on caffeine intake.** Eliminate caffeine for three or four days and bring it back in slowly. Keep your intake to one cup in the morning. Caffeine has a direct effect on our cortisol levels.
3. **Hang out with your girlfriends.** Studies show that close bonds between women increases the production of oxytocin, the feel-good hormone.
4. **Make love, alone or with another.** Orgasms help generate lots of health-boosting hormones.
5. **Supplements.** Consider the following supplements and/or botanicals: ashwagandha, phosphatidylserine, magnesium glycinate, L-theanine. (See also Chapter 7 for more on something called Cortisol Manager.)

Note: Remember to speak with your doctor if you have any medical conditions or are on any medications before taking new supplements.

LIVER 101: THE DETOXIFICATION SYSTEM

WHAT IS THE LIVER AND WHY SHOULD WE CARE?

1. The liver is the main filtration (or detoxification) system of the body.
2. The liver metabolizes our hormones. It's located on the right-hand side of your body under your rib cage. Gently place your hand there and notice it. Our livers convert excess estrogen into compounds that can be excreted through the bile and intestines and then out of the body.
3. Science shows us that eliminating estrogen safely can help women lose body fat and reduce our risk of cancer.
4. LOVE YOUR LIVER. Eat foods and drink teas that support its efficacy.

TOXINS, TOXINS, EVERYWHERE

I attended a medical conference a few years ago and learned this stunning piece of information: The average woman leaves the house each day wearing about 144 chemicals. If you pause for a moment and think about all the personal care products we use, and then consider how many chemicals each product contains, we start to see the bigger picture.

MARKERS OF AGING

INFLAMMATION 101

When it comes to inflammation, diets low in fiber and nutrients and heavy on carbs contribute to inflammation. Liver and kidney issues can also contribute to inflammation. (Note: Foods that contribute to inflammation are known as pro-inflammatory foods. I discuss this more fully in Chapter 5.)

I like to look at inflammation from the outside in. All of us, at one time or another, have experienced puffiness, stuffiness, bloat, and skin eruptions. Like an iceberg in the ocean, often we see just a small tip. But what's really going on is much deeper and pervasive and is often the root of health challenges and disease. We have to look at the cellular level. Perhaps it's an immune response to a certain kind of food, or you've flooded your system with sugar.

STRESS, SUGAR, AND INFLAMMATION

Be mindful of stress levels and how much sugar you consume. The less sugar you eat, the less insulin you need. The less insulin you need, the better your metabolism will be and less stress on your body. Less stress equals less inflammation. Less inflammation equals less cortisol being produced. Less cortisol being produced equals better health.

TELOMERES 101

TELOMERES ARE MARKERS OF AGING

Telomeres are the protective caps at the end of chromosomes (DNA). Telomeres resemble the caps on a shoelace and naturally get shorter as we get older. Eventually, telomeres get too short to do their job, causing our cells to age and stop functioning properly. Scientific research from Germany has shown practical ways to help promote the lengthening of our telomeres.

First and foremost, we can help lengthen our telomeres through exercise, specifically endurance exercise. Endurance activity has been shown to increase telomerase (the enzyme that lengthens the ends of telomeres with DNA building blocks) activity and telomere length, which are both important for cellular regeneration. Once the telomere completely depletes of telomerase, it eventually dies. The study found that forty-five minutes of continued running or endurance exercise three or more times a week corresponded with a spike in telomerase activity. This is good news as it puts power back in our hands. Yes, our actions *can* make a difference in how we age.

BODY SYSTEMS: WHAT YOU NEED TO KNOW

IMMUNE SYSTEM 101

Did you know that approximately 70 percent of your immune system is in your gut? Our guts may be the most important part of our bodies, especially as we age. Our guts are tied to the brain through the vagus nerve, which runs directly from the brain to the gut. So when you say, "I've got a gut feeling," you can rest assured that you are right on. Listen to those feelings. By improving your gut health you can support your immune system, overall health, and your intuition.

GUT HEALTH 101

The human microbiome, otherwise known as the community of bacteria (flora) that inhabit our guts and gastrointestinal tract, has an estimated 100 trillion microbes (bacteria). We have more microbiome than we do cells in our body.

A healthy gut can house over 1,000 different species of bacteria (though most studies show a healthy gut has about 300 different species).

Part of the microbiome's job is to make vitamin B12 and neurotransmitters, which are feel-good hormones. We need a healthy, diversified population of gut bacteria for our microbiome to perform its duties and contribute to our overall well-being. And we get healthy gut bacteria through diet, especially by eating plants.

Many chronic metabolic diseases are believed to begin in the gut. Current research shows that our microbiome can influence our metabolism, immune systems, inflammation, brains, and overall health and well-being. Everyone's gut microbiome is unique. But there are certain strains and combinations that are found in all healthy individuals. When the bacteria, yeast, and viruses are in balance in our gut, the rest of our body is in harmony too.

WHAT LEADS TO DYSBIOSIS, OR POOR GUT HEALTH?

Dysbiosis, or poor gut health, results from an imbalance in our gut flora caused by too few beneficial bacteria and an overgrowth of bad bacteria like E. coli and salmonella, yeast, and/or parasites.

Poor diet, unhealthy lifestyle habits, stress, and certain medications all affect the gut and can lead to a microbial imbalance and disruption of the microbiome. In turn, that can lead to a variety of health issues, especially inflammation, which is at the root of all chronic disease.

Bad bacteria have a mind of their own. We need a strategy for how to tame them. It's not as simple as using your willpower. These bad guys will do anything to survive—which even means leading you to eat sugar or junk just at the moment you've promised yourself you were going to stop. It's amazing how much power they have over our decisions. This is where we must become more conscious and awake and have a plan of action through diet, exercise, and supplementation.

HOW TO BUILD A HEALTHY GUT

Think of your gut as a field. To take care of the field, you need to fertilize it and make sure the soil is top notch.

We fertilize our guts by eating a variety of plants and/or by taking high-grade probiotic supplements to ensure that we have plenty of healthy bacteria. When our guts are fertilized and populated with a variety of healthy bacteria, we build immunity, fight disease, manufacture B vitamins, keep our weight in check, and support our best health.

LOVE YOUR BUGS!

To promote healthy bacteria, or what I like to call "the good guys," we start with diet and nutrient-dense food—like vegetables! What we put on our plate. How we digest our food. It all matters. Once you experience the positive benefits of healthy gut flora and a well-functioning gut, you feel more alive and energetic.

The gut has a tight barrier wall to protect the body from bacteria moving in and out. High levels of stress over time and some pro-inflammatory foods like gluten (for many) can make the wall weaker and allow tiny leaks to arise (think pinholes in a balloon). This is called intestinal permeability, which then allows gut bacteria (endotoxins) to enter the body. Now unhealthy bacteria are able to move in and out.

Current research suggests that these stress-induced changes may affect our brains and behavior as well. Evidence shows that certain hormones are made in the gut. Called gut peptides, they control the signaling between the gut and the brain. **When stress occurs, guts can produce inflammatory molecules. These guys disrupt brain chemistry and make many women more prone to anxiety and depression.** A stressed brain can inform the gut, and a stressed gut can inform the brain.

EAT FIBER. FIBER IS KING AND QUEEN. FIBER FEEDS THE GOOD GUYS.

When you eat fiber and it reaches the colon, it sends probiotics (good bacteria) into a feeding frenzy. (Think of this as a probiotic dance party!) The probiotics go to town, chowing down on their favorite food—fiber—and as a result (and gift to you), they produce postbiotics, or short chain fatty acids (SCFAs). These postbiotics, or SCFAs, are pretty magical.

Prebiotics (Fiber) + Probiotics (Bacteria) = Postbiotics (SCFAs)

WHAT ARE THE HEALTH BENEFITS
OF POSTBIOTICS (SCFAS)?

SCFAs have been shown to support a healthy inflammatory response throughout the body and lots of other health benefits in the gut and beyond, including improved learning and memory.

SCFAs correct dysbiosis by suppressing the growth of bad bugs; heal the colon wall by increasing proteins that help keep the colon wall intact; and support the immune system by helping it work properly and by playing a role in T-cell production, which keeps the immune system powerful and on track.

SCFAs also have a direct anticancer effect. They help regulate gene expression through enzymes known as histone deacetylases (HDACs). Multiple studies have shown that through their activity on HDACs, SCFAs are able to inhibit cellular proliferation. They actually stop dangerous cells, including cancer cells, in their tracks, causing apoptosis, or programmed cell death.

There are three kinds of SCFAs: butyrate, acetate and propionate.

1. **Butyrate** is made by the bacteria in our guts that ferment resistant starch and dietary fiber. It is the main source of energy and nourishment for the cells in the colon. Butyrate promotes colon health, decreases inflammation, and reduces our risk for colon cancer. Butyrate enhances insulin sensitivity and increases mitochondrial function. It also protects nerve cells and increases nerve growth by increasing brain-derived neurotrophic factor (BDNF). BDNF helps produce new brain cells and strengthen existing ones. Butyrate is essential for a healthy body and gut.

2. **Acetate** regulates the pH of the gut. It helps keep the gut environment stable and all the bacteria living in harmony. It controls appetite and protects against pathogens.

3. **Propionate** regulates inflammation and controls appetite.

The best way to get the health benefits of SCFAs is through the consumption of dietary fiber: fruits, vegetables, grains (in their whole form, not through flour), seeds, ground psyllium seeds, and nuts.

PREBIOTIC FIBERS: FOOD FOR THE PROBIOTICS

Prebiotic fibers are dietary fibers (Inulin, oligofructose, and fructooligosaccharides, or FOS) that help increase and feed the friendly bacteria already living in our guts. **Prebiotics include some very common foods like garlic, onions, bananas, oats, artichokes, and asparagus.** Most likely you already incorporate one or more of these three to four times per week in your diet.

Prebiotic fibers can favorably change the bacterial mix in the lower gut. They even help produce the hormones that control appetite and anxiety.

RESISTANT STARCH

Resistant starch is a carbohydrate that resists digestion in the small intestine and ferments in the large intestine. As the fiber ferments, it acts as a prebiotic—food for the probiotics.

Resistant starch helps create the SCFAs, including butyrate. Resistant starch can also help regulate insulin, promote gut health and help keep you feeling full longer.

Foods that contain resistant starch include:
- Plantains and green bananas
- Beans, peas, and lentils
- Whole grains and oats
- Cooked and cooled rice (cooled rice has more resistance starch than cooked)
- Cooked and cooled potatoes (cooking and cooling increases resistant starch; and boiled potatoes [try Japanese sweet potatoes!] also have a higher amount of resistant starch)

Eating these foods can positively affect our health. Because resistant starch doesn't digest in the small intestine, it doesn't raise glucose. Resistant starch boosts metabolism, helps manage blood sugar, and helps with insulin sensitivity. It contributes to digestive, brain, kidney, and eye health.

THE GAME-CHANGING POWER OF PROBIOTICS

Probiotics help digest food and assimilate nutrients.

You can't feed probiotics or good bacteria if you don't have any living in your gut, so to keep your gut flora strong, consider adding either well-tolerated sources of probiotic foods to your diet and/or a good professional-grade probiotic supplement.

Probiotic food sources include yogurt (dairy and plant-based), kefir, sauerkraut, tempeh, and kimchi. Probiotic foods help the flora in your gut reduce systemic inflammation, and they lower total cholesterol and LDL (or bad) cholesterol. They may also cause a reduction in blood pressure and boost our immune systems.

Most of us tolerate foods that contain probiotics well. The key when consuming foods containing probiotics is to look out for sugar. Sugar appears in nearly all packaged food we eat, including yogurt. It's certainly okay to have a sugary treat from time to time, but ultimately sugar is hard on the digestive tract and feeds the unhealthy bacteria in our gut such as yeast and fungus.

Further, we humans have a taste for sweetness and can quickly become addicted to sugar. So when you buy yogurt and kefir, for instance, look for unsweetened products or products sweetened with fruit and without cane sugar, as well as those made without the thickeners carrageenan or modified food starch.

Kefir is a cultured fermented beverage that tastes like yogurt. A super powerhouse food, kefir can have double the probiotics that yogurt contains. Kefir contains additional strains of good bacteria, and different kefirs contain different strains. It's fun and healthful to rotate brands. For a list of my favorite brands, visit marlynwellness.com.

Bone broth (or Grandma's chicken soup) is liquid gold. As you rebuild your body, it's important to lay a strong foundation, and you hit the jackpot with bone broth. Rich in collagen, vitamins, and amino acids that support the gut, bone broth is worth seeking out or making.

And bone broth is easy to make. You can use the carcass of a chicken like Grandma or any bones you wish. Cover them with water, add whatever savory you like, and simmer for hours until you've extracted all the goodness from the animal of your choice's bones.

Other ways to promote a healthy gut and good bugs:

- Intermittent fasting
- Mediterranean-based diet
- Professional-grade probiotics
- Vitamin D
- Omega 3s
- Berberine

FACTORS THAT AFFECT OUR FLORA:

- Antibiotics
- Prescription drugs, such as opioids, NSAIDs, PPIs, and statins
- Radiation/chemotherapy
- Sugar intake
- Bacteria in drinking water
- Pesticides in food
- Alcohol
- Heavy metals
- H. pylori (a bacteria that lives in the digestive tract)
- Stress
- Bowel transit time
- Allergies
- Gastrointestinal pH

MICROFLORA DISRUPTION LEADS TO:

- Leaky gut
- Non-alcoholic fatty liver
- Enteric nervous system imbalance
- Hormonal imbalance
- Systemic inflammation
- Immune issues
- Weight management issues
- Some cancers

HELPFUL TIPS

Many brain-related issues, such as anxiety, depression, and insomnia, can be traced back to the gut.

The Standard American Diet—known as SAD—decreases gut microbiome diversity.

Gliadin proteins (found in gluten) increase zonulin release, compromising junctional integrity in the intestinal tract and increasing gut permeability.

RADIANT TIP

EVERYDAY GUT HEALTH HABITS

Instead of thinking about it, we want to live it!

1. **Eat fiber at every meal.** Consume between 25–38 grams of fiber a day. Fiber increases the growth of healthy bacteria (especially lactobacilli, bifidobacteria, and prevotella) and also increases the diversity of species within the gut. Eat vegetables and prebiotic foods. (**Note:** Always consult with your physician regarding diet if you are faced with any specific gut/health challenges that require a modification of fiber.)

2. **Eat a variety of veggies.** Research shows that the single greatest predictor of a healthy gut is to include a diversity of plants in your diet. Keep loading up with fiber-rich foods and plants. If you tolerate fermented foods, which contain live microbiomes, well, add them to your diet. These foods include kimchi, miso, pickles, and raw sauerkraut.

3. **Try an ELIMINATION DIET.** This helps you identify and then avoid food triggers. (See Chapter 9 for more information.)

4. **Consider adding in a good, high-quality probiotic supplement** to your day.

5. **Hydrate!** Start your day with a glass of lemon water.

6. **Coffee** can benefit your gut with healthy acids like chlorogenic acid, polyphenols, and antioxidant compounds, which have prebiotic properties. Monitor your intake for a level that works with your sleep schedule.

7. **Exercise** helps you get more good gut bacteria. These good guys help you extract and unpack the nutrients in your food. Exercise also helps your body generate more SCFAs as well. But *how* isn't yet clear. This is an emerging science and clues to the gut-exercise connection are leading scientists and top researchers to continue to study this exciting field.

8. **Drink Grandma's chicken soup, aka BONE BROTH.**

9. **Limit** sugar, alcohol, stress, and medications. All affect the gut.

10. **Make time for FUN!** (This helps manage stress.)

STEP 6: HEALING THE AGING METABOLISM

We cannot solve our problems with
the same thinking we used when we created them.

– ALBERT EINSTEIN

The body knows how to heal itself and how to cleanse, regenerate, and repair itself. The body always seeks balance, and it also knows how to be nourished. It yearns for proper rest, hydrating liquids, and nutrient-dense foods that support it. That's why the first step on our healing metabolism journey is to acknowledge that our bodies are smart. They give us valuable feedback if we're awake and listening. Once we understand that *everything* we do—how we eat, move, sleep, and think—has a direct effect on our health and well-being, we can begin to make the necessary changes.

Creating a more efficient metabolism begins with better choices.

1. Diet
2. Exercise
3. Rest
4. Supplements
5. Intermittent fasting

WHAT IS INTERMITTENT FASTING?

INTERMITTENT FASTING 101

Intermittent fasting, or time-restricted eating, is a powerful lifestyle medicine tool that enables good health and sustainable weight loss. It also helps create cardio-metabolic resilience.

One of the most important steps we can take to increase our longevity is to take a break from food. Yes, that means intermittent fasting.

Intermittent fasting provides the body with metabolic rest that triggers the promotion of autophagy. Autophagy, which is part of the body's natural detoxification process, means self-eating. Our cells literally eat themselves and generate new ones.

Intermittent fasting is time-restricted eating or meal-timing. It helps you break out of fat storage mode, which many women face in midlife and in their menopausal years.

Intermittent fasting has been researched to help extend our health span, the years in which we enjoy optimal health.

Aging is complex. And we know that if we pay attention to our lifestyles, we can modify how we age. If you are overweight or obese, you are robbing yourself of health span. Obesity is widespread in the US. The latest studies (2017–2018) from the National Center of Health Statistics show that 41.9 percent of women are obese. If you have a body mass index (BMI) of greater than 30, you are considered obese according to the CDC (Centers for Disease Control).

Note: BMI is a tool, but it is not a diagnostic of the health of an individual.

Food lurks in front of us on every corner and in every convenience store and supermarket checkout too. For many of us, adherence to diets is so lousy. Believe me, I've tried them all (the grapefruit diet, the Scarsdale diet, calorie-counting diets, juice cleanse diets, etc.) and failed.

What has been researched to work best is this: Restrict food intake to an eight to ten hour window and allow a twelve to sixteen hour fasting window. It's free and impactful. Our ancestors practiced this. Our DNA evolved from this way of eating and living. The best news is that intermittent fasting is scientifically proven to improve insulin signaling.

Intermittent fasting flips on the metabolic switch. Instead of our bodies burning glucose, they burn fatty acids. When we fast, the body burns more fat. Fat gets mobilized into the cells to be used as energy.

Exercise while fasting is also beneficial. It creates mild to moderate stress on the body (called hormesis), which promotes adaptation where the body "adapts" and becomes stronger. Our adaptive homeostasis (or weight set point) declines with aging, and intermittent fasting and exercise effectively turns back the clock.

WHAT IS AUTOPHAGY AND WHY IS IT IMPORTANT?
AUTOPHAGY 101

Autophagy clears out the cellular junk. It's our body's way of eliminating damaged cells in order to regenerate newer, healthier cells. As we age, our cells gather a lot of junk, broken DNA, dead organelles, and oxidized particles, which can disrupt our cellular function and accelerate aging. By giving our bodies a break from constant feeding and digesting, our systems have the opportunity to regenerate and heal.

Our bodies are truly amazing and can do all kinds of exciting things. Giving ourselves the space and time to heal is a true gift.

Note: If you have a current health challenge, or are on any medications, please talk to your doctor before starting any fasting protocols.

HEALTHY AGING TIPS

RADIANT TIP

THE TRUE SECRET TO LOSING WEIGHT

Feeling better and getting our health in line is cultivating resilience and building our body's natural state of balance through the proper foods, lifestyle habits, sleep, mindset, and time-restricted eating.

RADIANT TIP

HOW TO BUILD YOUR BEST BODY

1. Reduce inflammation
2. Refocus your body's source of fuel/ nourishment
3. Intermittent fasting
4. Movement /weights

RADIANT TIP

KNOW WHAT'S BEST FOR YOUR BODY TYPE AND PLAY THE LONG GAME.

Break through the roadblocks that get in the way of living every moment in the radiant present. Enjoy the food you eat. Approach your challenges with an open heart and mind. Trust your intuition. Stay connected to your body and nature. Drink loads and loads of water. You can do this.

MICHELLE'S STORY

"From Flab to Fit!"

Michelle, fifty-seven, a mortgage broker in New York City and mother of two teenage boys, felt bloated and tired and had gained weight. For years, she lived a day in, day out, fast-paced lifestyle, and rarely took time to care for herself. Running from deal to deal, she usually ate on the go, grabbing sugary power bars, french fries, and deli sandwiches. Sometimes, due to her work schedule, she barely ate at all, only to come home famished and eat whatever was closest at hand—crackers, popcorn, and an array of junk food.

Throughout her adult life, Michelle had tried every quick-fix diet plan with no long-term lasting results. If she did lose weight, it would easily come back in a short period of time. Michelle attended a nutrition talk I gave in Great Neck, New York, in 2011. Afterward, she asked if we could meet and have a conversation. It became clear to her that she wanted to commit to a new way of eating.

Together we looked at her blood work and saw that she had high blood sugar and high insulin. Based on this, I concluded Michelle had insulin resistance, also known as weight resistance. I started Michelle on my 21-day transformational food plan and had her eliminate the pro-inflammatory foods she was consuming daily (wheat, refined sugars, and dairy.) I also recommended she eat more fresh fruits and vegetables, lean proteins, and nuts. In the span of five months, Michelle dropped twenty-five pounds, and as an added bonus, her husband dropped thirty!

Along with her weight loss, she lowered her blood sugar, insulin, and cholesterol and found herself with more energy than she had had in years, which she used to go to the gym and reclaim her body and physical strength. Michelle went from a size 10 to a size 4 and has maintained her weight loss for four years. No crazy diets, no funky pills or magic potions. Just healthy eating, a consistent supportive exercise plan, and an attitude that said, "YES I CAN!" If Michelle can do it, so can you.

A few thoughts on women, hormones, and menopause from David Allen, MD, an LA-based integrative and functional medicine physician and hormone expert:

- During menopause, we must look at a woman's **mind, mood, and behavior and balance her hormones.** For some women, bioidentical hormones are the key, replacing what was naturally in our bodies.

- We know **postmenopausal** women experience vaginal dryness and a loss of vitality and can be susceptible to dementia, cardiovascular disease, and osteoporosis.

- While moving through menopause and beyond, **diet is fundamental. Exercise** is important as well, especially resistance work. We lose muscle mass as we age. On average, we lose about 10 percent a year after age forty. Many times, women lose muscle and gain weight. The higher the muscle mass, the more calories burned. We must consciously build and replace the muscle we lose.

- Women, especially at midlife, are trying to do so much and wear so many hats, and we try to be A+ at everything. Our first job is to be healthy. Put on our own oxygen mask first. Watch our stress levels. Delegate. When we're in a chronic state of high stress, we produce more cortisol. High cortisol is going to break down muscle and accelerate aging. We must be honest with ourselves and acknowledge our limitations.

- **Foods that stimulate insulin,** like sugar, simple carbs, and white flour, should be cut out of your diet so you'll be ahead of the game.

CONGRATULATIONS, YOU DID IT!

We covered a lot here, and I acknowledge you for opening up your mind, diving in deep, and sticking with it.

Let's take a moment to pause, stretch, and breathe.

First, stand if you can, put your arms out to the sides, like wings on an airplane, and move them backward in a small circular motion five to ten times as you gently loosen your shoulders and continue to breathe in and out. Now reverse. Move your arms forward, in a circular motion five to ten times as you gently breathe in and out. Aaahhhh …

Next, sit comfortably (or continue standing) and put your arms up into the air as you clasp your hands together, and hold your index fingers (first fingers) out like you're shooting a love pistol into the air. With your arms extended, gently stretch to the right and feel the release on your left side. Hold that position for a few seconds, then bring your arms straight up, back to center. Continue grasping your hands, and gently stretch to the left, with your index fingers leading the way. Feel the release on your right side. Consider doing this two or three more times until your body feels more relaxed and open.

Now come back to a seated position with your arms gently by your sides and take a few more relaxing breaths. Focus all your attention on your breath moving in and out of your body. Deeply inhale as if you are smelling the most beautiful fragrant rose, ever. And again. Aaahhhh …

Did you have any new insights or revelations? Perhaps you want to open a journal and write them down.

Now that you're relaxed, let's learn about our blood.

Chapter 4

BLOOD DOESN'T LIE

"When a flower doesn't bloom, you fix the environment
in which it grows, not the flower."

– ALEXANDER DEN HEIJER

KNOW YOUR NUMBERS

What every woman needs to know about her blood tests. When it comes to our blood and blood work, we want to be empowered with the knowledge of what's going on inside. To do this, it's important to understand some basics about blood tests. I'm going to shed light on what to know and which tests to ask for.

We need to trust and become a partner with our doctors. We need to feel comfortable in their offices or on the phone with them. We also need to trust ourselves and become the CEOs of our bodies, because we are ultimately responsible for asking the right questions.

Blood tells a story. We want to test, not guess. Many traditionally trained doctors sometimes miss testing important areas that can give us deeper insight into our physical and emotional well-being. By testing a variety of markers, you and your doctor will get a larger picture of what you need to become healthy and strong. Your knowledge will help you understand how to address symptoms like fatigue, weight loss resistance, or thinning hair.

Our doctors want to help us, and we are there to understand the whole picture of our bodies and how they work and to gain a broader perspective of our health. *This* is how we step into the role of CEO. And to do this effectively, we need to understand the basics of our blood.

RADIANT TIP

TEAM UP WITH YOUR DOCTOR

At this stage of life, more than ever, we need to take responsibility for our life. We want our doctor to be a collaborative person who works with us. Talk to your doctor. Challenge them. Ask them to show you the study if their opinion goes against something you believe in deeply. We want to feel well-equipped to promote our maximum health.

RADIANT TIP

If your doctor won't order the following tests, consider going to WellnessFx.com or MyMedLab.com to get them done.

TOP TESTS FOR WHOLE BODY HEALTH

Remember: Getting the right tests for YOU is empowering!

Blood Panel: It's best to draw blood before 9:30 a.m., after you have fasted for the night.

VAP cholesterol: This full cholesterol panel includes subtypes of LDL and HDL plus lipoprotein.

Cholesterol is an essential substance for the body. The body needs cholesterol to make hormones, vitamin D, and certain substances that play a role in digestion.

Cholesterol is a waxy, fat-like substance found in our body's cells and in many of the foods we eat (beef, chicken, turkey, and other animal proteins).

Here are the types of cholesterol:

- **High Density Lipoprotein (HDL):** This is usually referred to as good cholesterol, or healthy cholesterol. HDL helps to remove unhealthy cholesterol from your body.

- **Low Density Lipoprotein (LDL):** Too much of this cholesterol can lead to a buildup of plaque in your arteries.

- **Very Low Density Lipoprotein (VLDL):** This type of cholesterol can also promote too much buildup of plaque in your arteries.

- **Triglycerides:** These are a specific type of fat. High triglycerides may mean you have excess fat in the body or may be at increased risk for type 2 diabetes. For some, high triglycerides may signal you are consuming too many calories, especially from sugar, refined grains, and processed foods that contain hydrogenated fats. Smoking and excess alcohol consumption can also lead to high triglycerides.

It's important to understand the difference between good cholesterol and harmful cholesterol. We want our cholesterol to be light, fluffy, and buoyant. The challenge comes when our cholesterol is thick, hard, and dense. This type of cholesterol has a tendency to build up in the arteries and block blood flow. Just because your cholesterol numbers come back high does not mean there's a problem.

A VAP (vertical auto profile) test is an excellent way to see what type of cholesterol your body is producing. Once you have the knowledge, there are ways through diet, lifestyle, and supplementation that have the potential to shift the cholesterol to light and fully if that is what's needed. Cardio activities and foods high in omega 3, like wild salmon and sardines, can be excellent in supporting the manufacturing of good HDL cholesterol. On occasion, our cholesterol levels are impacted by genetics, although many times lifestyle changes can improve your numbers.

RADIANT TIP

FOOD THOUGHTS
FOR HEALTHIER CHOLESTEROL

1. **Add In Plant Sterols:** nuts (especially walnuts), seeds, whole grains, olive oil
2. **Limit Saturated Fats:** butter, fatty animal protein, lard
3. **Select Lean Proteins:** lean beef, chicken, turkey
4. **Include Soluble Fiber:** oats, whole brown rice, ground flaxseeds

HERE ARE MORE RECOMMENDED TESTS TO CONSIDER:

- CBC w/ platelets (CBC stands for complete blood count)
- CMP or comp metabolic panel, which includes fasting glucose and fasting insulin
- Hemoglobin A1c
- Homocysteine
- Vitamin D OH25 + Vitamin D3
- CRP or C-reactive protein, which looks at inflammation in the body

WHO SHOULD GET A BLOOD TEST?

Most adults, particularly women, and those experiencing fatigue and poor mood.

RADIANT TIP

FASTING BLOOD GLUCOSE

A fasting blood glucose of less than 100 mg/dL is considered normal. But most functional medical doctors agree that optimal numbers range from 70–85mg/dL. This gives you a cushion.

A1C: AN IMPORTANT BLOOD TEST
(BLOOD SUGAR)

A1c is a blood test that provides information about a person's average levels of blood sugar over the last three months. I often recommend this test to my clients to gauge how well they are metabolizing sugar. The A1c is excellent in detecting the possibility of insulin resistance. An HbA1c test measures the percentage of red blood cells saturated with glucose. The higher your A1C, the higher the estimated average blood glucose. In addition to diabetes, a high HbA1C marker may also increase your risk of Alzheimer's disease and cancer, potentially making the test a good predictor of overall longevity. Ideally you want your HbA1C to be 4–5.7. Lower is better.

1. A1c is also referred to as hemoglobin A1c or HbA1c. Where testing blood sugar might vary from day to day, A1c gives us a bigger picture about what's going on over time.
2. A1c test does not require fasting so it can be done any time of day.
3. A1c tests can vary in results, though in the big picture they are quite reliable as a tool to assess overall health and especially blood sugar health.

Many people feel like they are destined to the genetic hand they've been dealt. Genes are important, and it's key to know your family history. It's empowering to have awareness around the diseases, health challenges, and genetic mutations that run in your family.

Let's say your family has a propensity for blood sugar imbalances, type 2 diabetes, or easily gaining weight. With this basic knowledge, we can become aware that we may be facing a high sensitivity to refined sugars and high-carbohydrate foods. We may learn that our cells are more sensitive to metabolizing glucose and as a result lean toward wanting to store glucose as fat. Once we understand where we are *now*, we can begin to change the playing field going forward by making new choices centered around a higher protein, lower-carb eating plan, more exercise, personalized supplements that target blood sugar support, and lowering our overall sugar intake.

THYROID 101: THE MASTER GLAND

HOW THE THYROID WORKS AND WHAT IT DOES

The thyroid is the master gland. Butterfly-shaped, it sits in the front of the neck, just below the Adam's apple. Thyroid hormones play vital roles in regulating the body's metabolic rate, heart and digestive functions, muscle control, brain development and function, and the maintenance of bones. Each of our cells has a receptor for thyroid hormone. You can compare the thyroid gland to an engine in a car. Just as a car needs an engine to run smoothly, the body needs the thyroid gland to run smoothly.

The thyroid produces a hormone called thyroxine, known as T4. T4 gets converted into triiodothyronine, or T3, the active form of thyroid hormone. Once converted, T3 is readily available for cellular uptake. Think of T3 as the gas that runs the body.

On occasion, some of us have trouble converting T4 into T3. This can happen for a variety of reasons, including poor gut health, because the gut is one of the areas where T4 is converted into T3.

In addition, some T4 gets converted into reverse T3, an inactive form of T3. T3 and reverse T3 can also compete with each other for uptake at the cell receptor site. Because reverse T3 is an inactive form of T3, if it is taken up by the cell, the cell won't get the energy it needs from the active T3.

When the reverse T3 number is high, it may also indicate high stress levels at play and/or high cortisol levels (stress hormones).

WHEN YOUR THYROID ISN'T FUNCTIONING PROPERLY, YOU MAY EXPERIENCE:

- Brain fog
- Slow bowels/constipation
- Hair loss
- Hormonal imbalances
- Weight loss struggles

For many, thyroid challenges are underdiagnosed. Most traditional physicians look for normal ranges within a thyroid blood test. Normal levels may vary due to various labs. Thyroid numbers may not always reveal a clear picture. We want to look at symptoms too. From a functional medicine perspective, for optimal health, we aim for thyroid numbers to be in high normal ranges (again, levels may vary due to various labs). The majority of functional medicine doctors and practitioners are highly trained in the area of thyroid health. If you are at all concerned about your thyroid, talk to your doctor, and consider arranging for the following tests.

Thyroid panel:
- TSH
- Free T4
- Free T3
- Anti-TPO (thyroid antibody to check for autoimmune Hashimoto's)
- Anti-thyroglobulin (thyroid antibody to check for autoimmune Hashimoto's or autoimmune Grave's disease)

If you are feeling tired and stressed, include:
- Reverse T3

RADIANT TIP

FOODS FOR THYROID

Seafood, shrimp, kelp, nori, seaweed, dulse, sea salts (good source of natural iodine)

Avoid excess gluten, fluoride, and chlorine, which have been studied and are shown to have an adverse effect on the thyroid. Brazil nuts are especially good for the thyroid as they contain selenium, which the thyroid uses to convert T4 to T3.

NOTE: If you experience unexplainable weight gain or loss, chronic fatigue, cold intolerance, hair loss, forgetfulness, constipation, and are feeling generally depressed, you may benefit from having a thyroid panel done.

RADIANT TIP

AT AGE FORTY-FIVE, REQUEST A BASELINE HORMONE PANEL

At forty-five, it's especially helpful to get a baseline hormone panel. This shows you where your hormone levels are before menopause, so you can begin monitoring your body as it changes. After menopause, it's beneficial to get an updated blood test once a year. This allows you and your doctor to watch for hormonal changes that may be contributing to weight gain, mood swings, and sleep challenges and take corrective action if needed. Corrective action may look different for each person. For some it may include bioidentical hormones. For others it may include dietary and lifestyle changes, and/or the addition of targeted herbs, teas, or tinctures.

The hormone panel includes:

Sex hormones: estradiol, progesterone, and free, bioavailable, and total testosterone

FSH (follicle stimulating hormone)

LH (luteinizing hormone)

DHEA-S (dehydroepiandrosterone sulfate): if overweight add leptin, the fat storage hormone

Sex hormone binding globulin

Adrenal Panel: cortisol, DHEA

Pregnenolone

Total cortisol

If you feel extra tired and you can't shake your lethargy, you may want to consider testing for Epstein-Barr virus antibodies and/or Lyme disease.

RADIANT TIP

BLOOD TESTS + FUNCTIONAL MEDICINE = KNOWLEDGE

When reviewing and interpreting blood panel results, it may be beneficial to work with a functional medical doctor, health practitioner, or trained certified nutritionist who is versed in functional medicine. For assistance in locating a qualified practitioner in your area, check out The Institute for Functional Medicine: https://www.ifm.org.

Remember, knowledge about our precious bodies puts control back in our hands. Many of us are afraid to know our bodies' inner workings. But with the right knowledge and confidence in ourselves, we can understand our unique relationship with our health. Each choice we make, can and does have a direct outcome on our greater health and wellness.

DIANA'S WELLNESS JOURNEY

Part 2

After a few weeks of in-person coaching sessions, Diana was following her new protocols, feeling better and more in control of her food and snack choices. She was still struggling with weight loss, which was causing her to feel pretty frustrated inside. I suspected something might be off with her hormones and/or glucose numbers and recommended she see her physician to get a blood test.

Diana saw a functional medicine doctor and had a panel of tests. The results came back within a week and revealed that she had high insulin, high A1C, low thyroid, and low testosterone—

all contributing to a hormonal imbalance and inability to release weight. Her functional medicine doctor prescribed a low-dose thyroid replacement, and he and I agreed that it would be helpful to add in a few key supplements to help support her blood sugar levels and regulate her insulin. Supplements included alpha-lipoic acid, berberine, and a multivitamin with chromium. I also recommended that Diana stay committed to her lower-carb, low-glycemic, anti-inflammatory eating plan, exercise plan, and nightly twelve to thirteen hour intermittent fasting schedule.

Finding out what was at the root of her inability to shed weight uncovered pieces that were extremely helpful on the journey. At this point, Diana was in good spirits and was hopeful that with continued determination and focus, she could lose the weight she desired and feel better overall.

At one of our first coaching sessions, I taught Diana one of my favorite mantras, STICK-TO-ITIVENESS—meaning stay diligent and no throwing in the towel, no matter what! Although she had been really frustrated at times, Diana stuck with the mantra and stayed on the path instead of giving in to the voice in her head that told her to give up.

Coming up... Diana hits new strides in her mind/body adventure and shares her formula (in Chapter 7) for creating a day of wellness, including simple steps that helped her build an easy, attainable structure and ongoing success.

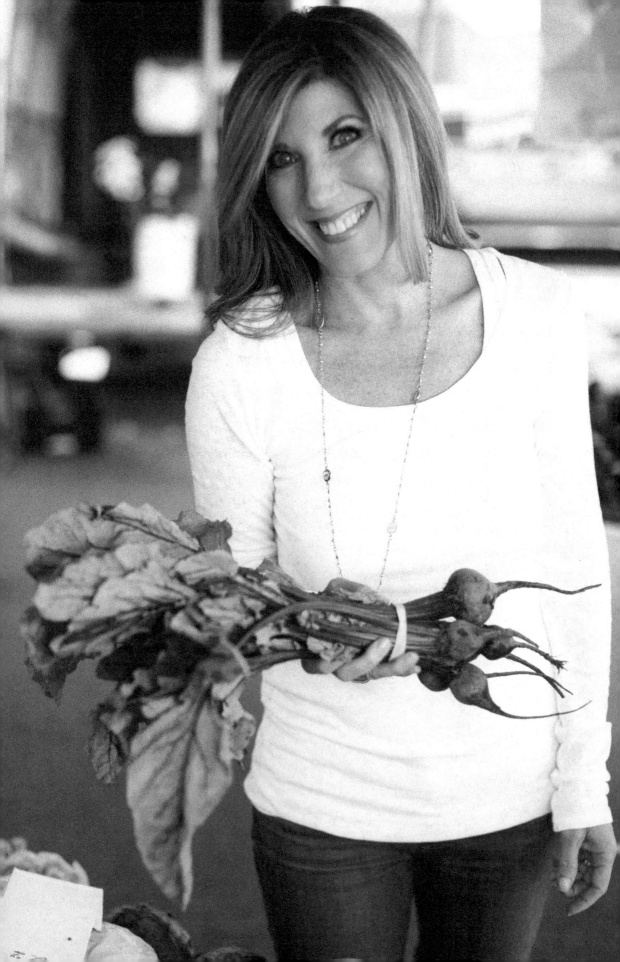

Chapter 5

NEXT-LEVEL NUTRITION

"Between stimulus and response, there is a space.
In that space is the power to choose our response.
In our response lies our growth and freedom."

– VICTOR FRANKEL

Going to a new nutritional level requires growth. And our actions matter. When the going gets hard, as it will, I'm here to say, "Stick to and through it." Because a few months from now, the things that felt really hard will become routine—and *that* becomes the new normal.

When we're up-leveling our lives, we want to look at our habits, core beliefs, daily routines, the people we live and socialize with, and our environments.

In this chapter, we look at our food. We'll also look at our habits, beliefs, and daily routines. Each day, the most powerful decision we can make regarding our health is what we put on our plates. Eating should be a joy. But so many of us are confused about what the right diet is for us, what the labels on our food mean, what to buy, and how to prepare it. We've also grown confused about sugar and the underlying causes that can lead to addiction.

SO, LET'S TALK ABOUT FOOD.

Food is pleasure. Food is medicine. Food is nourishment. Food is energy. Food is family. Food is love.

BUT, FIRST AND FOREMOST, FOOD IS INFORMATION.

While food is meant to bring us great pleasure, it's important to remember that food is more than the calories it contains. Food gives your cells instructions. Each ingredient has its own code. And with every bite, food can upgrade your biological software or downgrade it.

Compare 250 calories of broccoli to 250 calories of soda. Your body will obviously receive very different information from the broccoli and that has a huge effect on your metabolism, your brain chemistry, your hormones, your immune system, and your microbiome, the bacteria that run the gut and rule the body as a whole.

Every single bite of food changes your biology in real time. It is the most powerful drug on the planet. Like that beautiful tart-crisp first apple of fall, full of antioxidants, vitamins, and phytonutrients, food is loaded with ingredients that fuel the direction of your energy and immunity.

Food has a role in gene expression, our biology, and creating health and disease. Food tells the cells what to do. It has the ability to turn on genes and cellular functions that activate healing measures and protect our cells from further damage.

Common diseases and conditions can be improved by food. The body has enormous ability to respond quickly to the food we eat to fix ourselves and our brain. I watch these miracles happen every day in my own body and in my nutrition practice. Eating the wrong food can lead to disease. Eating the right food for your body can lead to a healthy life.

Think about your beautiful body and mind, your blood flowing through your veins, your gorgeous brain and its ability to not only process information but to create. Think of the luxury of a good night's sleep and the gift of a robust and satisfying sex life. They are all affected by the food you eat.

DISCOVERING FOOD THROUGH THE LENS OF FUNCTIONAL MEDICINE

I've spent more than thirty years studying nutrition and over twelve years practicing as a clinical nutritionist. And I am always learning. In 2007, when I discovered functional medicine, I adopted its simple tenet: Food is medicine.

I try to be my best client, looking at medical studies, attending medical conferences, taking what I've learned and applying it to my own diet. I've learned about supplements and the proper way to take them. And I've learned to rest so that my body can integrate not only the food I take in, but also manage the little stresses that make up a normal day.

Functional medicine has given me a blueprint and framework for understanding how the food I eat affects the life I live. From that first introduction in 2007, I have never looked back. It is my guiding light. My roadmap to health.

Below are some basic principles I've learned through my own studies and through functional medicine that have helped me shift my body and mind to one of health, energy, and vibrancy.

BEYOND RADIANT FOOD PRINCIPLES

1. **Eat real food.** Take a look at your pantry. If your shelves contain chemical-infused packaged foods and unhealthy snacks, throw them away. You wouldn't sprinkle BHT or methylcellulose on your beautiful veggies, so why would you tolerate it in packaged food?
2. **Add more vegetables to your diet.** Eat every color of the rainbow. Increase the number of plants you eat daily to 70–80 percent of your total intake.
3. **Eat animal products that are good for you and good for the planet.** If you're

going to eat meat and can afford it, choose animals who were raised or fed a diet of grass or real plants without chemicals, antibiotics, and feed (like GMO corn and soy products) designed to make them fat fast! Think about the quality of the life of the animal. Grass-fed beef is a great source of protein and is higher in omega 3 fats, antioxidants, and amino acids too. If your budget doesn't allow for higher-priced animal protein, limit your intake and splurge when you can. Buy a whole organic chicken. Cook the meat, then simmer the bones to make broth.

4. **Eat small fish.** These fish, like sardines and anchovies, are a great source of omega 3 fatty acids, which are brain food. Many larger fish like swordfish, tuna, and sea bass have higher mercury levels. It doesn't mean you shouldn't enjoy a beautiful grilled swordfish steak. Just be mindful. Avoid farm-raised when you can.

5. **Add nuts and seeds.** If you're not allergic to them, nuts and seeds are nutrient-dense and contain high amounts of healthy fats and zinc, which is good for our immunity, skin, and overall well-being. Consider trying nut flours in baked goods.

6. **Eat beans and legumes.** If you're worried about weight gain after eating a plate of rich and delicious refried beans, try smaller, non-starchy beans and legumes like lentils and peas.

7. **Add whole grains.** The best grains for managing your blood sugar are whole brown rice, millet, quinoa. Grains grow in the ground, and in some cultures they are considered a "grounding" food, meaning they take you from living in your head to being back in your body. Eating the right grains can create a sense of calm, especially after a jam-packed day. Be mindful of portions. Watch out for rice flour, corn flour, and wheat flours. While these flours can produce delicious treats, when they are ground into fine powder, they quickly turn into sugar and you run the risk of spiking your blood sugar.

NOTE: **If you are vegan,** it's easy to consume lots of starch and high-sugar foods such as pasta and bread. Too many carbs can contribute to weight gain, insulin resistance, and blood sugar imbalances. Focus on more nutrient-dense foods, including nuts and seeds. Consider taking spirulina to add B12 to your diet. Hemp seeds, often overlooked as part of our daily diet, are rich in protein and provide omega 3, 6, and 9 fatty acids, which are brain and skin food!

BLISS POINTS

WHAT'S THE FOOD INDUSTRY GOT TO DO WITH IT?

In the early part of my career, I worked in the food industry and have some behind-the-scenes insights.

First, the food industry deliberately hires scientists to create bliss points. Bliss points are the place where taste, texture, and mouthfeel meet. And those scientists are invested in creating projects that hit that biological trifecta.

Foods designed to target our bliss points literally light up certain parts of our brain, robbing us of free choice as we perceive it. Eating that bag of nacho cheese tortilla chips will make your brain chemistry wacky and knock your metabolism off its routine. It tricks the bacteria in your gut so that you crave carbohydrates and sugar. And guess what? You have the makings of an addiction.

For most of us, this cycle of addiction starts when we are young. Remember Saturday mornings in front of the TV watching cartoons and knocking back a bowl of Sugar Pops or that strawberry Pop-Tart? Or perhaps your family welcomed you home after school with a glass of boring milk made delicious with a heaping tablespoon or more of Nestle Quik, the delicious sugary chocolate powder spiked with artificial ingredients. Oh, but it tasted so good.

We were naive then, as were most of our parents. Unless you had very food-conscious parents or caretakers who cooked a lot of homemade simple meals and fed you fruit and nuts as snacks, you and your brain may have been hijacked by big food and fast food too.

These habits run strong and last into our adult years until we wake up one day, or read a book, or get a health diagnosis, or have an experience with a healer, physician, or practitioner that shows us the real power of food and how the wrong foods can wreak incredible havoc on our health and well-being.

IN ORDER TO RECLAIM OUR FOOD AND PALATE POWER...

1. **We must name the problem and awaken to the steps** we must take to change our way of eating. We want to eat more beneficial ingredients. We want to use food to heal. We want to avoid toxic environments.

2. **We must have clear pathways and understanding to take action.** We eat three times a day (or more), and each time we eat, we get to vote with our fork. What are we eating? What are we drinking? What are we buying? It all matters!

Imagine if ... we started to choose whole foods and shift our diets.

We have the power. What we've given away, we can reclaim. Perhaps you already eat healthy foods but would like to explore the best diet for your body and lifestyle. And if you're not eating as healthy as you would like, trust me, you can change. We can all change. It's our choice.

3 STEPS TO PULL BACK THE CURTAIN ON OUR FOOD

STEP ONE: READ LABELS

Many companies have a way of labeling ingredients that is confusing to us, the consumers. It's worth your time to familiarize yourself with the labels of your favorite foods. Here are some of the more common ingredients and food additives to be aware of:

Natural flavors: Many of the chemicals that make up natural flavors fall under a category called Generally Recognized As Safe, or GRAS. An estimated 3,000 chemical food additives fall into this category. Yet it doesn't mean that these chemicals have been widely studied by the FDA. Food companies are not required to disclose the ingredients that make up a "natural" flavor. And there can be upwards of 100 ingredients in one "natural" flavor, including preservatives, solvents, and other substances, which are defined as "incidental additives." Additionally, food manufacturers are not required to disclose whether these incidental additives come from natural or synthetic sources.

According to the US FDA code of Federal Regulations, natural flavors are substances extracted from plants or animal sources: spices, fruit or fruit juice, vegetable or vegetable juice, edible yeast, herbs, bark, buds, roots or plant material, and dairy products (including fermented products, meat, poultry, seafood, and eggs). Natural flavors can be obtained by heating or roasting the animal or plant material. Natural flavors are complex mixtures created by specially trained food chemists called flavorists.

Many of these natural flavors may also contain a glutamate by-product, which is MSG. These chemicals (glutamate by-products) are known as excitotoxins. Excitotoxins are chemicals added to food to make it tastier. Excitotoxins cause brain cells to become very excited and can trick our brains into overeating, setting up a pattern of addiction. Unless the label lists the exact ingredients in the natural flavor on the package, be mindful that these natural flavoring ingredients may come from natural sources that have been altered in a lab.

Carrageenan: This is a thickener. Joanne K. Tobacman, MD, has published multiple peer-reviewed studies on the biological effects of carrageenan and believes that all forms of it are harmful. She has found that exposure to it in the amounts contained in processed foods causes inflammation in the body. That's concerning, since chronic inflammation is a root cause of many serious diseases, including heart disease, Alzheimer's and Parkinson's diseases, coronary artery disease, and cancer.

Maltodextrin: This is a thickener. Maltodextrin is high on the glycemic index, meaning that it can cause a spike in your blood sugar. It's safe to consume in very small amounts, but those with diabetes should be particularly careful.

MSG (monosodium glutamate): This is a flavor enhancer that often shows up in canned food like soups, processed meats, and Chinese takeout. It can cause:

- Headache
- Flushing
- Sweating
- Facial pressure or tightness
- Numbness, tingling, or burning in the face, neck, and other areas
- Rapid, fluttering heartbeats (heart palpitations)
- Chest pain
- Nausea
- Weakness

Researchers have found no definitive evidence of a link between MSG and these symptoms, but they acknowledge that a small percentage of people may have short-term reactions to MSG. Symptoms are usually mild and don't require treatment. The only way to prevent a reaction is to avoid foods containing MSG.

SUGAR

There are over fifty names for sugar. And it is a primary ingredient in many packaged foods. If sugar is one of the first three ingredients, I recommend putting the package down and making a healthier choice.

Examples:

- Agave nectar
- Barbados raw sugar
- Barley malt
- Beet sugar
- Cane sugar
- Corn syrup
- Date sugar
- Dextrose
- Evaporated cane juice
- Fruit juice concentrate
- High-fructose corn syrup
- Honey
- Molasses
- Sucrose

Sucralose: This is derived from sugar, but not absorbed by the body. Animal studies link sucralose to negative effects on the bacterial environment in the gut. However, human studies are needed. Sucralose is added to a lot of diet food and sugar-free products.

Be aware of foods containing sugar: Refined carbs, made from processed grain flours, get metabolized and converted quickly into glucose and rapidly raise blood sugar. This includes candy, cakes, donuts, pastries, cookies, ice cream, frozen yogurt (usually loaded with chemicals!), white bread, bagels, rolls, pretzels, pasta, crackers, and cereal. Remember to read labels.

Highly processed foods and commercially packaged foods: When you buy processed foods and read the ingredient list, look for things your grandmother wouldn't recognize or are impossible to pronounce.

Sugar-sweetened drinks: These include regular soft drinks, fruit juices, sweetened iced tea, lemonade, Gatorade, sports drinks, vitamin water, mixers, spritzers, spirits, wine, that double pumpkin latte you just ordered.

Trans fats: Hydrogenated or partially hydrogenated oils are usually added to products to help with mouthfeel and to keep the foods shelf-stable. Processed seed and vegetable oils include soybean, sunflower, corn, canola, and vegetable oils. They are cheap, less expensive oils and most are made in a lab. Some even use formaldehyde. These oils have a tendency to create high amounts of inflammation in the body.

BECOME A SMART CONSUMER. READ ALL FOOD LABELS and ingredients, even on food labeled as healthy, organic, or all natural.

RADIANT TIP

EXAMPLES OF HEALTHIER CHOICES

If you'd like a touch of sweetness in your food, here are some better options:

- Monk fruit
- Honey, raw, unrefined
- Manuka honey
- Coconut sugar
- Lucama
- Maple syrup, unrefined
- Date paste
- Figs

RADIANT TIP

SEVEN STEPS TO OVERCOMING SUGAR ADDICTION

1. Avoid refined sugar.
2. Include lots of whole fresh foods in your diet.
3. Avoid junk food.
4. Eat fish three times a week or take a fish oil supplement.
5. Stay hydrated. Drink a quart of water a day (pure or in herbal tea).
6. Minimize your intake of coffee, caffeinated teas, and alcohol.
7. Eat at least five servings of antioxidant-rich fruits and vegetables a day.

BRENDA'S WELLNESS STORY: KICKING THE SUGAR HABIT

Brenda, fifty-two, a mom, activist, and leader in her community, was highly addicted to sugar. It was constantly sneaking into her life through her daily food choices, girlfriend lunch celebrations, and Saturday night desserts. She especially loved sweet, sugary chocolate! On a positive note, Brenda has always been a huge fan of exercise. Growing up as a competitive gymnast, movement was a key part of her everyday life and kept her slim and fit. As she entered her forties, she found herself eating too much sugar, especially during any stressful period she came up against.

When I first met Brenda in 2007, I taught her about the power of reading labels, which ingredients to avoid, and introduced her to my 21-day transformational food cleanse as a way to boost her metabolism and tame her sugar cravings. Additionally, I upgraded her favorite foods to ones made up of healthier ingredients and designed a delicious, nutrient-dense chocolate morning smoothie loaded with superfoods and healing ingredients like ashwagandha, maca, reishi mushroom, and MCT oil to start her day off with energy and pleasure.

As the days and weeks passed, Brenda gained back control over her sugar cravings and began making more conscious choices. Now sugar-sweetened desserts were an occasional treat on a Saturday night or a few bites here and there when she was out with the girls. During her wellness journey, Brenda lost nine pounds, inspired her husband (who lost weight and became super healthy too!), family, and friends, and created healthier habits to support her best self as she moved into her fifties.

STEP TWO: AVOID PROBLEMATIC FOODS

PROBLEMATIC FOODS AND FOODS THAT COULD BE CAUSING US PROBLEMS

When I meet with my clients, the most common challenges they share are:

- Inflammation*
- Acid indigestion
- Bloat and gas
- Weight gain
- Sleeping issues
- Belly fat

*Inflammation is the body's attempt at self-protection to remove harmful stimuli and begin the healing process. Inflammation can be good or bad, depending on the situation. It is part of the body's immune response. Infections, wounds, and any damage to tissue would not be able to heal without an inflammatory response. As we get older, we become more at risk for chronic, sustained inflammation. As mentioned above, and in Chapter 3, food is one of the top contributors to inflammation in the body.

TOP FIVE INFLAMMATORY FOODS TO CONSIDER AVOIDING OR REDUCING:

1. **Gluten:** The word gluten is the Latin word for *glue*. Gluten is the protein found in wheat and provides elasticity to foods. Gluten can also make us fat. When ingested, it can trigger a response in the body and brain that causes immune overreaction and increased appetite. This can hook us into overeating. Much of the wheat grown in the US is dwarf wheat, GMO, and/ or sprayed with glyphosate (a toxic weed killer), which is hard for the body to break down. It wreaks havoc on our gut lining by creating tiny pinhole-like openings where food can leak out and cause the body and immune system to create a reaction that can lead to bloating, belly aches, and immune system malfunction.

   Look for organic bread made with nut (almond) or coconut flour. These do not turn into sugar quickly. Be mindful of rice flour and potato starch–based breads that may spike your blood sugar.

2. **Dairy:** For many, dairy is difficult to digest. Adding to the challenge with dairy are the number of animals raised with hormones and antibiotics. If you're going to have dairy, choose raw, hormone-free, and grass-fed whenever possible. Lean toward goat or sheep milk because the A1 casein (a protein) from cow's milk is hard to break down for most humans. Goat and sheep have an A2 casein, which is easier for many to digest.

   Chemical and sugar-free yogurts (without additives or sugar substitutes) and kefir-based products can be good for some, especially as a way to populate our good gut bacteria. It's a matter of running an experiment on yourself, as we'll do in the cleanse chapter, by leaving dairy out of your diet for a short time and then bringing it back to see how you feel.

3. **Processed soy:** Processed soy is not a whole food in its whole form. It has been taken out of its whole food form and has been processed in a laboratory to become a different form. An example of this is isolated soy. This is found in many protein powder products, bars, and vegetarian products made to simulate meat, like veggie hot dogs or fake chicken tenders. Processed soy for many can contribute to health challenges and inflammation. When choosing soy products think organic tofu, fermented miso, unsweetened, non-GMO organic soy milk, or tempeh.

4. **Refined sugars:** We've discussed sugar above, though let me share a bit more here. Refined sugars have been stripped of any kind of nutrition. Yes, refined sugar brings pleasure in small doses, but in larger quantities, it depletes the body and triggers and accelerates the aging process. Let's return to insulin resistance. When our cells are bombarded with sugar, they have a lowered response to insulin and glucose. Sugar overload is at the root of a lot of our health challenges. If you're going to sweeten your food, consider using dates, a small amount of coconut sugar, raw honey, or a bit of 100 percent maple syrup.

   NOTE: If you are a diabetic or someone who is highly sensitive to any refined sugars, be mindful of all sugars. You may consider using monk fruit or lucama, as these do not spike blood sugar.

5. **Industrial oils (vegetable and seed):** Canola, corn, cottonseed, soybean, and sunflower oils are linked to a higher rate of inflammation. They can also cause problems with insulin and leptin (the hormone that tells the body when it's full). They wreak havoc on our metabolism and contribute to making us fat. Tip: Be mindful of where you dine out. Many restaurants use these oils in their cooking.

INFLAMMATORY CHEMICALS IN YOUR FOOD

I could write another book on food additives and preservatives, a hot button of mine! For the sake of keeping things simple, I'm going to share my biggest concerns. With that, if something interests you, I encourage you to dig further and tap into the research.

1. **Food colors:** FD & C Red 40 and Yellow 5 and 6 are a few examples. They seem innocent, though unless the food color on the package specifically says "plant-based," they are usually made in a lab and can be detrimental to our overall health. Red 40 and Yellow 5 and 6 contain compounds (benzidine and 4 aminobiphenyl) that research has linked with cancer. Research has also associated food dyes for some children to be associated with allergies, irritability, and aggressiveness. Be aware that many over-the-counter medications and prescription meds contain artificial dyes and colors. Check labels.

2. **Preservatives:** Consider citric acid. It can contain mycotoxins, which for some can be an irritant and trigger asthma symptoms.

3. **Sodium:** This is found in many processed meats and rotisserie chicken and is used to plump it and make it juicy.

4. **Stabilizers:** These include BHT and BHA and keep food shelf stable—otherwise food would rot.

5. **Gellan gum:** This is a thickener. Look for it in plant-based milk and plant-based coffee creamer. Be mindful, as this can cause gut/intestinal irritation

BE YOUR OWN FOOD DETECTIVE

Clients often come into my practice when their otherwise robust health has been disrupted. They come to me with allergies, or they are experiencing mood swings, headaches, bloating, and skin eruptions. And many times these distressing conditions seem to come out of nowhere.

I ask them to remember the last time they felt vibrant and healthy. What changed? Was there a new food they added that started making them feel ill? Have they gone through a stressful period, hormonal shifts, a traumatic incident, financial challenges? Did they recently travel overseas? Did they recently undergo home construction, which may have contributed to the release of toxic mold or exposed them to fumes from glues, varnishes (think kitchen cabinets or new carpets), or other unhealthy chemicals?

When you look back and examine the before and after of events and experiences in your life, you will have a clearer picture about what's going on in your body.

RADIANT TIP

ARE FOODS TRIGGERING YOUR SUFFERING?

The next time you have a headache, sleepless night, or poor digestion, it's worth taking a look at what might have triggered it. Look at the foods you last ate and the way you handled your stress. The clues are everywhere. If you regularly suffer from bloating, gas, indigestion, and insomnia, there's a high likelihood you will find connections to the foods you eat.

STEP THREE: INCORPORATE HEALING FOODS AND ADAPTOGENS

The body is smart. Our job is to support and to collaborate mind/body wisdom. We do this by putting the right nutrients in and letting it do its job.

"Let food be thy medicine and medicine be thy food."

– HIPPOCRATES

FOOD IS MEDICINE

My personal philosophy has always been to look at food as medicine and to use it to improve my health and emotional state. Since my breast cancer diagnosis in 2015, I've taken my interest in food to a whole new level. When I eat or teach my clients to eat, I focus on maximizing the nutritional content of each meal. For example, I'll add a dash of turmeric to a shake or latte for an extra immune-boosting ingredient. I'll put ½ teaspoon of ashwagandha in a smoothie, tea, or tonic for better stress reduction and mood support. I'll sprinkle a dash of dulse seaweed (high in iodine) into my soup or salad for enhanced detoxification and better thyroid and breast support. Once you start to learn more about these healing superfoods, this becomes fun and a bit like playing your own nutritional alchemy game.

METHYLATION ADAPTOGENS (POLYPHENOLS)

There's an exciting area of growing research focusing on the powerful components of certain plants that have the ability to enhance healing, boost immunity, and support our internal tumor-suppressor genes. These foods are known as methylation adaptogens and have been shown in studies to favorably alter genetic expression. (How amazing is that!)

They are loaded with antioxidants, flavonoids, and concentrated polyphenols (potent plant medicine), which help our bodies adapt to our environment, internally and externally. Just as some foods cause havoc in the body, methylation adaptogens can favorably upgrade our internal environment and alter genetic expression.

Top ten polyphenol methylation adaptogens to support immunity and positive genetic expression:

1. **Curcumin:** Found in turmeric
2. **Sulforaphane:** Found in cruciferous vegetables like broccoli and cauliflower
3. **Luteolin:** Found in celery, thyme, and chamomile tea and may be helpful for reducing inflammation in the brain
4. **Lutein:** Spinach, kale, and yellow carrots and beneficial for eye health
5. **Lycopene:** Tomatoes, especially cooked
6. **Rosmarinic:** Rosemary, basil, sage, thyme
7. **Quercetin:** Red onion and apple skins, green tea, red grapes

8. **EGCG:** Green tea and white tea
9. **Genisten:** Soybeans
10. **Apigenin:** Parsley, artichoke, grapefruit, onions, oranges, chamomile, and celery

RADIANT TIP

Eat one serving of your choice of methylation adaptogens a day. Of course, you can always eat more and mix and match as you choose.

HEALING SPICES

Spices, salts, and herbs support longevity, better metabolism, better breast health, better beauty, and reduced inflammation. Below are my top ten favorites. Try them on your favorite foods or bring in others you enjoy as well.

1. **Turmeric:** Anti-inflammatory and boosts immunity.
2. **Cinnamon:** Boosts metabolism, balances blood sugar, and is antiviral. (Ceylon is my favorite due to its purity and the fact that it contains active compounds including cinnamtannin B1, which has been shown to improve fasting blood glucose levels in people with type 2 diabetes.)
3. **Himalayan pink salt:** Contains up to 84 trace minerals and is beneficial to your health. Celtic sea salt is another great salt that is loaded with minerals from the sea.
4. **Cayenne:** Revs up your metabolism. Capsaicin (a constituent in cayenne) may control certain types of pain. It tricks the body into feeling fuller by stimulating the brain's satiation receptors. It's also good for breaking up mucus and stagnation in the body. It's especially helpful during the change of season when moving from winter months into spring.
5. **Ginger (fresh and powdered):** Anti-inflammatory, antioxidant powerhouse.
6. **Fresh nutmeg:** Warming to the body and beautiful for the senses.
7. **Dulse seaweed:** High in iodine, which supports thyroid and breast health.
8. **Cardamom:** Warming to the body and helps with blood flow. Ancient

medicine lists cardamom as a powerful aphrodisiac and especially good for men's sexual health and performance. Let's hear it for the cardamom spiced smoothie or latte for your special honey!

9. **Rosemary:** This is anti-bacterial.

10. **Cumin:** Supports digestion and improves antioxidant absorption.

RADIANT TIP

HERBS AND SPICES ARE WELLNESS WARRIORS!

Healing herbs, mineral salts, and gorgeous dried spices are the unsung heroes of the food world. Think of them as your personal wellness assistants breaking up mucus and inflammation in the body, supporting blood flow, revving up your metabolism, and heightening your overall health and well-being. They give flavor to food and are powerful cancer-fighting, anti-inflammatory, and disease-prevention warriors. Sprinkle on salads, stir-fries, and in soups. Add to smoothies, shakes and tonics. Explore, experiment, and play.

ADAPTOGENS: MEDICINAL MUSHROOMS AND HERBS

Adaptogens are roots and herbs known for their healing, toning, and strengthening abilities. Adaptogens are helpful for blood, body, bones, and organs. Many have been used for centuries in Chinese and Ayurvedic medicine. Today we are lucky to find them conveniently available in powders, pills, and tinctures at our favorite health food markets. (See resource guide.)

Adaptogens
- **Ashwagandha:** A plant with a full spectrum of healing properties that may: soothe anxiety, support sleep, and tonify the immune system. (In Chinese or herbal medicine, *tonify* means to increase the available energy or strengthen.)
- **He shou wu:** Blood and longevity tonic. Regular consumption may help to tonify and nourish blood, hair, skin, nails, and sexual center. Help improve stamina. Enhance immune function. Promote red blood cells.

- **Pearl:** Used for improving beauty and mood and stimulate collagen.
- **Astragalus:** Used to boost immunity.
- **Bacopa:** A potent neuero-protective elixir that may support mood, mental clarity, and overall brain function.
- **Maca:** Promotes energy, hormone balance, and enhanced libido.
- **Shatvara:** A potent elixir that may help with hormone balance and whole body rejuvenation. Its cooling calming effect may help alleviate hot flashes during menopause.
- **Schisandra berry:** Promotes glowing Skin and supports libido and memory.

Medicinal mushrooms are known for their antiviral, anti-inflammatory, and healing effects on the body.

Medicinal Mushrooms
- **Reishi:** Promotes immunity, calm, and longevity
- **Cordyceps:** Promotes energy, libido, and stamina
- **Lion's mane:** Promotes brain health, focus, and immunity
- **Chaga:** Promotes longevity and immunity and slows aging
- **Maitake:** Promotes immunity and is antiviral
- **Turkey tail:** Promotes immunity and is antiviral

RADIANT TIP

ADAPTOGENIC BEAUTY BOOST

Consider adding adaptogens and/or medicinal mushrooms to coffee, tea, lattes, smoothies, oatmeal, or snacks for a brain, body, beauty, and/or blood sugar boost.

NOTE: If you are on medication or have specific health challenges, consult your health practitioner or doctor for guidance.

As we move forward, let's take a look at all that we've learned and apply it in a doable, inspired way. We'll look at simple strategies and fun ways to incorporate the basics of eating well and living mindfully into our everyday lives.

PART II:

HEALTHY, HAPPY, AND HORMONALLY BALANCED

Chapter 6

MARLYN'S METHOD FOR MIDLIFE!

I know once people get connected to real food, they never turn back.

– A L I C E   W A T E R S

MY MOTTO

"I believe in clean, whole eating. I believe in living a life of passion, pleasure, and joy. I believe in an all-encompassing approach to reach your wellness goals. There are no quick fixes or fad diets. It's always about progress, never perfection. Through small incremental shifts, implemented over time, you will achieve long-term sustainable change."

It's easy these days to get caught up in a feast of overwhelm, especially when it comes to diet and what to eat. Here, I'm excited to share my cornerstones of simple daily practices when it comes to choosing how and what to eat. No need to be 100 percent keto, paleo, plant-based, or etc. (Do these only if you want to.) You can choose to be keto-ish, paleo-ish, or vegan-ish. Truthfully, there's no right or wrong. The foundational principle is to have simple rituals and clear practices that can help you navigate how to feed your body and choose the foods that are right for you. When you crowd out fake foods and bring in a lifestyle based on your inner wisdom and real, whole foods, you will reduce the stress that often accompanies a feeling of: "What the heck should I eat?" Below are some of the key ways you can begin to get clear about how to create a life of health and choose a way of eating that is not only simple, but that also works for you.

NOTE: I've taken some of the best concepts I learned throughout my more than six years in formal mindfulness training classes (including Mindfulness Basics, Mindfulness-Based Stress Reduction, Mindful Self-Compassion, Mindfulness for Parenting, and Mindful Eating) and infused them here and throughout the book.

MY THREE-STEP APPROACH
TO EVERYDAY EATING:

1. Intuitive eating
2. The ACE formula: Add in, Crowd out, Elevate up
3. Eat a rainbow of colors

INTUITIVE EATING

One of the great joys in learning to trust your intuition to navigate how and what to eat is that you will no longer be a slave to diets. Instead, you'll become a thriving intuitive eater.

As intuitive eaters, we use *internal* cues rather than *external* cues to guide our food choices. We approach food (and lifestyle) choices from a place of self-care, permission, and acceptance of our bodies rather than self-control, deprivation, and weight shaming.

BUT WHAT EXACTLY IS INTUITIVE EATING?

We are born intuitive eaters. Somewhere along the line, this gets lost: shame, judgment, society, and social media can all be factors. We end up losing touch with our internal cues and eat according to external cues instead: the latest fad diets, calorie counts, body weight, rules regarding "good" or "bad" foods. Intuitive eating is more about letting these external cues go and listening to our bodies.

Think back to a time when you were sick. Most likely you were looking for lighter fare or healing food like chicken soup, crackers, or toast, instead of a big steak, a glass of wine, and french fries.

Intuitive eating is more an art than a science. Since our bodies are always changing, our eating patterns change from day to day too. The more you step forward and tune into your internal cues, the better you get at it. This takes practice, just like playing an instrument or learning to speak a foreign language.

Your body and your gut are smart. They know. And the more you listen, the more you'll hear what they are telling you. Your gut is programmed to tell you when it's full. Get quiet. Listen for the cues. And don't forget the satisfaction factor: that moment when you push your plate away and are ready to face the world.

INTUITIVE EATING = MAKING FOOD CHOICES WITHOUT EXPERIENCING GUILT

Now that we've gotten quiet, let's listen to our beautiful bodies. Perhaps you need more raw food, or cooked food, or a bit more fruit, vegetables, or a warm cup of soup. When we get quiet, talk to our bodies, and listen for the answers, we hear things we may have never paid attention to before. As we put those answers into practice, we'll build our self-esteem and confidence. We'll learn to differentiate between emotional and physical forms of hunger, fullness, and satiety. And many times, in doing this, we learn that what we need to satisfy and satiate us isn't even food. Maybe it's more joy, play, sex, adventure, connection, a deep conversation with a good friend, or getting outside in nature.

Once we develop our intuition, it will become a guiding voice that allows us to make better decisions with food and in our lives.

INTUITIVE EATING TOOL KIT

1. Your body is smart and knows what it needs for optimum health. Listen to it.
2. Cravings leave clues. What are your cravings? Perhaps there's a nutrient you need.

3. Reject diet culture. Embrace a healthy lifestyle instead.

4. Honor your hunger and respect your fullness cues. Discover the satisfaction factor.

5. Practice mindful eating.

6. Challenge the harsh internal voice and the food police in your head.

7. Approach things with curiosity instead of judgment.

8. Be more compassionate with yourself.

9. Make peace with your body.

10. Honor your feelings without using food.

11. Honor your health and well-being.

12. Exercise and feel the difference. Drop the unreasonable food rules: the good/bad, the should/shouldn'ts.

13. Rid yourself of guilt and anxiety around food.

14. Enjoy the pleasure of eating.

"Food is meant to nourish our bodies and bring pleasure,
not solve our problems."

HEAL YOUR RELATIONSHIP WITH FOOD, BECOME MORE MINDFUL.

Along with the practice of intuitive eating, we practice mindfulness. Through mindful eating, we will celebrate the food on our plate, we become aware of all the components that are influencing our decisions about food—emotions, physical cues, timing, access—and we will do this without judgment. We will simply observe.

ON BECOMING MORE MINDFUL:

1. In difficult moments, allow yourself to feel whatever comes up for you without using food to numb or avoid the discomfort.

2. Honor your health. Instead of grabbing a donut or bag of cookies, choose foods you enjoy that nourish you.

3. Trust your body. Drop the food rules. If you have a guilty pleasure, enjoy a small portion of it. (Use the Three-Bite Rule in Chapter 11.)

4. Listen to your body. It will tell you when it's truly hungry.

5. Take pleasure in meals. Enjoy the process of shopping for food, cooking, and eating.

BEYOND RADIANT MINDFUL EATING HABITS

The environment in which we prepare and eat our food makes an important contribution to the nourishing influence food has on the body. By paying attention to a few simple principles, you can help your system extract the highest levels of nourishment from everything you eat.

- **Sit down to eat in a relaxing, settled environment.** Turn off the TV and put your phone away.

- **Eat freshly cooked meals** whenever possible.

- **Create a beautiful tablescape:** Light a candle, arrange flowers, use lovely plates.

- **Reduce the amount of ice-cold foods and drinks you consume.** They put out your digestive fire. Think of digestive fire as the heat that digests our food. This is similar to a furnace that burns charcoal or wood, only with our digestion, we need all the proper nutrients to be extracted from the food and assimilated into the body for energy, vitality, and life force. The term digestive fire stems from Chinese and Ayurvedic medicine. It's a fascinating theory, and I highly recommend learning more about it! According to these 5,000 year old ancient medicine modalities, very cold drinks and too much cold food can constrict blood flow in the digestive system and slow enzymes, which in turn causes stagnation and a slower metabolism. If we're not digesting our food (or our life experiences) properly, we are oftentimes left with discomfort, pain, constipation, etc.

- **Engage in thoughtful conversation or silence.**

- **Eat at a moderate pace.** Chew your food. Put down your fork in between bites.

- **Aim for twenty-minute meals.** This will support weight loss and better digestion. Studies show that eating quickly may cause people to overeat, and as a result, they gain more weight over time. After a meal, your body releases the hormone leptin that lets your brain know it's full. It takes about twenty minutes for the signals to get to the brain. By slowing down, you give your brain time to receive the signals.

- **Wait until one meal is digested** before eating the next.
- **Leave ⅓ to ¼ of your stomach empty** to aid digestion.
- **Sit quietly for a few minutes after your meal.** Take a walk, if you can.

A FEW MORE THINGS TO CONSIDER:

1. If you're eating take-out food, put it on a beautiful plate or dish. Set the stage to engage fully with your eating experience.
2. Take the time before meals to appreciate the food in front of you: color, aroma, texture, meal prep. Be in gratitude to whomever made it. Note the flavors and textures.
3. Take a bite and chew!

RADIANT TIP

MINDFUL HABITS

To change our condition, mindset, or situation, we must shift our habits. We begin by becoming mindful (or aware) of what we eat. When we eat. With whom we eat. Whenever possible surround yourself with people and places that uplift you. And when that is not possible, bring those people and places to mind.

ACE FORMULA
(ADD IN, CROWD OUT, ELEVATE UP)

In 2016, I was invited to speak at the Fourth Annual Student Conference for Integrative Medicine (ASCIM) at UCLA. The event was organized by the integrative medicine students. One hundred fifty people filled the room: high school students, undergraduate and graduate medical students, health professionals, faculty, and members of the Los Angeles community.

The nutrition section was titled, "What Should I Eat? A Talk with Nutrition Experts," and featured Felicia Yu, MD, speaking from an Eastern perspective; Rammohan Roa, MD, presenting from an Ayurvedic perspective; and myself, sharing a Western perspective. I wanted to make it easy for all attendees to think about their daily food choices and decided to create the acronym ACE. Because who doesn't love to ACE a test or work project? So, let's ACE our nutrition and healthy habits too!

ACE stands for: Add in, Crowd Out, and Elevate Up. It's an easy-peasy way to think about your food.

1. **Add In:** Farm fresh foods and nourishing meals and snacks. Whenever possible, choose hormone-free lean meats, wild-caught fish, free-range eggs, organic seasonal fruits and veggies, low-sugar fruits like berries and green apples, healthy fats like olive oil, avocado oil, and hemp seed oil, raw and sprouted nuts and seeds (almonds, walnuts, and pumpkin seeds), and a variety of healing herbs and spices like ginger, garlic, turmeric, oregano, cinnamon, and rosemary.

2. **Crowd Out:** Begin to release additives, chemicals, pesticides, and refined sugars in processed and packaged foods. Take an inventory of your pantry. Look where additives are hiding: in your coffee drink, salad dressings, sauces, canned goods, and on your sandwiches.

3. **Elevate Up.** Swap up to healthier selections. Bake a batch of homemade cookies with the best ingredients, instead of buying packaged, chemical-laden cookies. Choose organic coffee instead of regular coffee that may be sprayed with pesticides.

EAT THE RAINBOW
HOW TO EAT THE RAINBOW

The key to eating a healthy diet is simple; Eat your colors. So go ahead, make a salad. Fill it with deep greens, yellows, purples, reds, oranges. Add herbs and spices for flavor and additional healing properties. The more informed you are about the benefits of each food you put into your body and the positive chemical reactions you'll experience, the more you'll find that you no longer need willpower to avoid unhealthy choices—because your brain is changing along with your body.

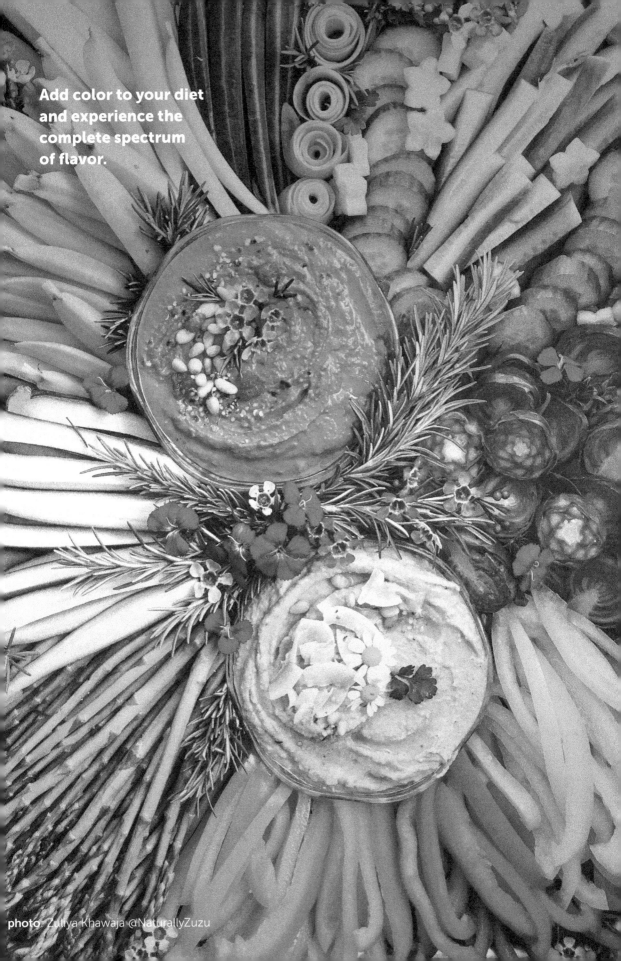

Add color to your diet and experience the complete spectrum of flavor.

Colorful fruits and vegetables contain powerful antioxidants and phytonutrients that can help protect your energy and support your cellular health. Consider this: When you bite into and chew broccoli, its enzymes, myrosinase, combine with our saliva to create sulforaphane, which is a powerful antioxidant that fights cancer. A cup of broccoli a day is amazing for immunity, detoxification, and healthier estrogen metabolism.

Think of eating a rainbow as an insurance policy for your greater health and wellness.

Every color in the vegetable kingdom—or, as I like to call it, queendom—represents a different family of healing compounds.

When we eat a rainbow, we are adding disease-combating nutrients (polyphenols), vitamins, and minerals to our diet. And don't forget, many of us eat with our eyes. Deep rich colors can add both beauty and fun to our plates.

HEALTH-BOOSTING, BEAUTIFUL, VIBRANT COLORS TO ADD TO YOUR DAY:

Red: Toss antioxidant-rich raspberries, strawberries, goji berries, or pomegranate seeds into your salads or oatmeal. Pomegranate seeds are especially rich in phytonutrients, tannins, and anthocyanins that can lower blood sugar and reduce blood pressure. An apple a day, rich in pectin and fiber, may indeed keep the doctor away. Add roasted beets to salad or kidney beans to a rice dish. Pecans and sprouted buckwheat also count as reds, as well as juicy tomatoes. Dark sweet cherries add a boost of flavor to any smoothie or snack, and are loaded with D-glucarate (a powerful cancer fighter) and support better melatonin production for a peaceful night's rest.

Orange/Yellow: Thick creamy, roasted butternut squash, sweet potatoes, and pumpkins all contain lots of beta-carotene. Oranges, tangerines, almonds, and cashews make wonderful snacks. Enjoy carrots, orange and yellow peppers, nectarines, peaches, and apricots, which are great snacks and a nice addition to salads. Grate a knob of ginger and toss it in your stir-fry, smoothie, or tea. Add a turmeric latte to your afternoon break, or enjoy it as a wind-down drink before bed.

Green: Chlorophyll (energy from the sun!) gives greens their rich hue. Sauté or roast broccoli, asparagus, kale, spinach, and/or bok choy. Squeeze lime on an avocado and you've got a great green snack. For crunch, toss pistachios or pumpkin seeds into a mixed green salad and top with a drizzle of extra virgin olive oil. Other delicious options include kiwis and green grapes. For a metabolic boost and some cancer-fighting goodness, enjoy a matcha latte in the morning instead of your regular brew or as an afternoon pick-me-up.

Blue/Purple: In Chinese Medicine, blue and purple foods keep blood vessels healthy. Sprinkle chopped dried figs or plums in a salad. Mix blueberries and blackberries into grain-free cereal. Roast purple eggplant or shiitake mushrooms and serve as a side dish. Flaxseed, seaweed, black beans, black quinoa, and wild rice are all in this family as well.

White: Toss some pine nuts into a salad or create your own mixed-nut adventure. Cut up a luscious pear and top with almond butter for a sweet, high-fiber treat. Onions, garlic, and cauliflower are loaded with sulfur for better detoxification, gut health, and beautiful hair, skin, and nails. Use them as ingredients in a side dish, or toss into a stir-fry. Mushrooms pack a punch when it comes to vitamin D. Mix and match the various varieties for flavor, texture, and taste. The whole white family of veggies are delicious drizzled with a little olive oil and roasted until sweet.

RADIANT TIP

ON SEX

The adage goes, "You are what you eat," and what you eat shows up in life *and* in the bedroom—in your energy, your mood, and your presence. A beautiful variety of colorful fruits and vegetables contributes to your most radiant, healthy self—the "girl with the glow." Eating a rainbow of colors has the capacity to elevate our energy and heighten our senses. Your body is your vessel. It's designed to give pleasure and receive pleasure too. As women, we often forget that piece—our pleasure. So feed your temple well and allow your energy to flow, in and out of the bedroom. You are worth it!

A FEW MORE THINGS TO CONSIDER:

- **Eat food in its whole form.** The best foods come right from the earth. If you're buying packaged foods, look for simple ingredients. One or two and try your best for no more than five ingredients. There are, however, always the exceptions, like Trader Joe's eggplant hummus, which is eight ingredients: chickpeas, eggplant, sesame tahini, lemon juice, garlic, water, sea salt, pomegranate juice (no fillers or additives!). Another example might be a gluten-free bread made from eggs, almond meal, coconut flour, apple cider vinegar, honey, baking soda, and sea salt (no fillers or additives!). Then of course, there's packaged nuts and seeds or jars of coconut or nut butters that may have pure vanilla bean, cocoa, and sea salt added for flavor. Again, these are all foods in their whole form or juiced form for flavor and color. Avoid chemical additives, preservatives, fillers, and fake foods.

- **Know your ingredients.** If there's an ingredient in your packaged food and you have to look it up, or your grandmother wouldn't know it, you probably want to avoid eating it!

- **Choose fresh, seasonal foods, preferably organic, when possible.** If organic is too expensive or unavailable, you can consider buying what's in season and/or frozen organic food, which is usually less expensive than fresh and is for the most part picked at the height of the season. Do your best to rinse and wash your fresh produce thoroughly with a veggie wash or Dr. Bronnner's soap, available at most markets.

- Choose wild over farm-raised, and grass-fed and pasture-raised, when available.

A POWERFULLY PORTIONED PLATE

Now let's tie this all together to create a **powerfully portioned plate.**

WHAT DOES A HEALTHY PLATE OF FOOD LOOK LIKE?

Look at your plate. Divide it in half. Now, take one of those halves and divide it again. Ideally half of your plate should be filled with vegetables, one quarter with protein, about the size of the palm of the hand or a checkbook, and the remaining quarter filled with either grains (I prefer gluten-free) or a starchy vegetable. Starchy veggies are also referred to as slow carbs because they are carbohydrates (energy) that break down and burn slowly over time. On top of your salad or vegetables, add a small amount of healthy fat like ¼ of avocado or 1–2 teaspoons of extra virgin olive oil. If you cook your vegetables in olive oil or other healthy fat, that counts too.

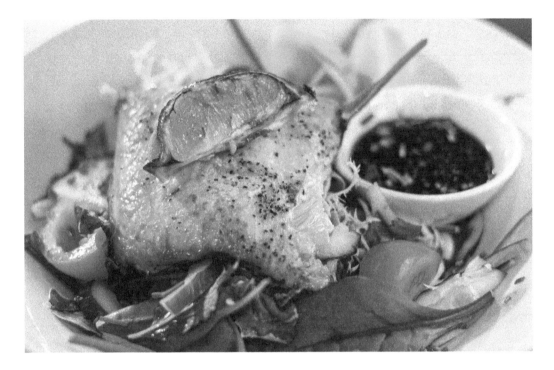

MEDITERRANEAN ANTI-INFLAMMATORY DIET

- **Grains and starchy carbohydrates:** You want to look at the total load of sugars you eat in a day. Starchy vegetables, such as potatoes, or grains, like rice, break down into sugar (glucose). A good rule of thumb is to keep grains to approximately ½ cup per meal and potatoes to one small potato or half of a large one. These foods add healthy pleasure, but if quantities are too large, they are hard for many women to metabolize and this may lead to weight gain. Personally, I love the sweet and satisfying taste of caramelized roasted sweet potatoes. But when I eat them, I follow my quarter-plate rule. I remind myself that the key to long-term health lies in the portions I choose to consume and how much physical activity I've added to my day.

- **When it comes to protein,** there are different ideal sources for different people. We can choose either animal or vegetable protein. If we choose animal, it's worth buying grass-fed beef, organic meats, and organic or cage-free chicken. Take time to do your research. In the case of processed or in a ready-to-go cooked rotisserie chicken, sodium and sodium nitrates are often injected to plump the chicken and make it juicier. Read labels.

- **Choose wild-caught fish.** One of the worst foods out there is farm-raised salmon. Unless specifically advertised, farm-raised salmon are usually fed a corn-based diet, given antibiotics, and fed pink dye to simulate the color of their flesh when they are in the wild. Have you ever seen a salmon swim through a cornfield? I also recommend that you buy frozen wild as opposed to fresh farmed. There are companies where you can order online and get wild or ocean-raised products, so do your research. And buy things on sale in season. For instance, if your favorite fish is in season, buy a little extra, freeze it, and use it over a period of time.

- **Eggs** are an excellent source of protein for many, and farmer's markets are great places to buy eggs. Look for omega 3, non-grain feeds, no antibiotics, and pasture-raised.

- **For vegetarians, vegans, and those of us who like to eat plant-rich meals, beans and lentils are a great source of plant-based protein.** I recommend soaking beans/lentils overnight. If you use beans from a can, buy BPA-free and rinse off the starch. Beans have a protective agent (phytic acid) on them that's hard for most of us to digest, and also they're a carb-protein mix so they can cause gas for a lot of us. Soaking dried beans breaks down phytic acid and helps with digestion. When cooking beans, adding kombu, a form of seaweed, also helps break down the sugars and makes them more digestible.

HOW MANY CALORIES SHOULD I EAT?

CALORIES 101

A calorie is a measure of energy. But let's ask ourselves: When is one calorie different from another calorie? A good place to start is to understand what calories are made up of and what those calories are doing to our blood profile over time. Here, we can take a deeper look at cellular health and what the calories we consume are contributing to or depleting from our cells.

Instead of using our food to store fat, we want to use food for fuel. We work toward this by becoming more mindful of our portions and filling our plates with *lots* of vegetables and low-glycemic (low-sugar) foods and small amounts of quality protein and healthy fats to support our daily nutritional needs.

Think blood sugar–balancing meals and snacks, instead of calories. It's okay to be mindful of calories. Though better yet, learn good portion sizes for your body type. It's time to take a more relaxed healthy approach to eating. Use the guide below to look at what a good day of food might be for you.

DAILY FOOD GUIDE

In 2009, after completing an intensive training program with Metagenics in Orange County, California, I became a certified **FirstLine Therapy®** Lifestyle Educator. Metagenics is a leader in educational research and evidence-based nutrition and personalized lifestyle medicine. The First Line Therapy program is based on a Mediterranean diet lifestyle and is rooted in the philosophy of food first. This means food is our first line of defense when it comes to creating health and avoiding chronic disease.

The sample day guide below is based on the First Line Therapy principles with my own small modifications added in. I created it to help you navigate serving sizes and portions. Keep in mind this is a guideline. Depending on how many servings you choose, it is based on a 1200–1400 calorie Mediterranean, low-glycemic eating plan. If you are hungry, have extra protein and veggies. You can tweak and tailor this plan to your day and your body. Some days you may want less food, some days more. Use this guideline as a starting place or foundation for your healthy eating lifestyle.

SAMPLE DAY

- 1 plant-based protein shake (if you choose to drink a shake): Some examples are: rice, pea, hemp, or pumpkin seed protein powders.
- 2–3 servings of protein (approximately 4 ounces per serving): Consider 2 servings if you are having a shake.
- 1 serving of dairy/dairy alternatives (8 ounces serving milk or plant-based milk, 6 ounces yogurt or plant-based yogurt, 2 ounces cheese or plant-based cheese)
- 1 serving of legumes/beans (1/2 cup per serving)

- Unlimited non-starchy veggies (such as lettuce, cucumbers, broccoli, cauliflower, onions, mushrooms, jicama, etc.)
- 1 starchy veggie (½ cup of carrots or beets, ½ cup of butternut squash, ½ sweet potato)
- 1–2 servings of fruit (1 small apple, 1 cup of berries, 1 pear, etc.)
- 1 serving of nuts (1 tablespoon of almond or nut butter, 10–12 almonds, 8 whole walnuts, small handful of pumpkin seeds, etc.)
- 1 serving of grains (½ cup of brown rice or quinoa, 1 slice of millet bread, 5–8 gluten-free or whole grain crackers)
- 4 servings of healthy fats or oils (a serving is 1 teaspoon olive oil, ¼ small avocado, or 6 olives)

NOTE:

- If you want more nuts, have fewer legumes.
- Be mindful of fruit in your shakes as part of your daily servings.

WHAT DOES A HEALTHY DAILY SERVING LOOK LIKE?

CONCENTRATED PROTEIN (meat, fish, chicken): 2–3 servings

1 serving = approximately 150 calories

Serving size: 3-4 ounces cooked, or as indicated

- Meat: poultry, and fish should be grilled, baked, or roasted; fish may also be poached.
- Eggs: 2 whole, or 3 egg whites plus 1 whole egg
- Fish: shellfish, 3–4 ounces fresh, or 3/4 cup canned in water
- Poultry: chicken or Cornish hen, turkey
- Lamb: Leg of lamb, lean roast
- Beef: buffalo, venison, elk
- Tofu: 5–6 ounces, or 1 cup fresh
- Tempeh: 3 ounces or 1/2 cup, 1/3 cup seitan
- Veggie burger: 4 ounces

LEGUMES/BEANS: 1 serving

1 serving = approximately 110 calories

Serving size: ½ cup cooked, or as indicated

- Beans: garbanzo, pinto, kidney, black, lima, cannellini, navy, mung, soy
- Bean soups: 3/4 cup
- Hummus: 1/4 cup
- Split peas, sweet green peas, lentils

DAIRY ALTERNATIVES: 1 serving

1 serving = approximately 80 calories

Serving size: 6 ounces, or as indicated

- Almond or soy milk, unsweetened: 8 ounces
- Hemp milk, plain: 6 ounces
- Unsweetened coconut milk: 8 ounces
- Yogurt (plant-based): 6 ounces

NUTS AND SEEDS: 1–2 servings

1 serving = approximately 100 calories

Serving size: as indicated

- Almonds or hazelnuts: 12–14 or 1/2 ounces
- Coconut, unsweetened grated: 3 tablespoons
- Pine nuts: 2 tablespoons
- Pistachios, sunflower, pumpkin, or sesame seeds: 2 tablespoons
- Walnut or pecan halves: 8–10
- Nut butter: 1 tablespoon made from above nuts

NON-STARCHY VEGETABLES: minimum of 5 servings

1 serving = approximately 10–25 calories

Serving size: 1/2 cup, or 1 cup for raw greens

- Artichokes, asparagus, bamboo shoots
- Bean sprouts, broccoli sprouts, or other sprouts
- Bell pepper or other peppers
- Broccoli, broccoflower, Brussels sprouts

- Cabbage (all types), cauliflower
- Celery, cucumber
- Chives
- Eggplant, garlic, green beans
- Greens: bok choy, escarole, Swiss chard, kale, collards, spinach, dandelion, mustard, and beet greens
- Leeks, kohlrabi
- Lettuce/mixed greens - romaine, red and green leaf, endive, spinach, arugula, radicchio, watercress, chicory
- Mushrooms, okra, onions, radishes
- Salsa (sugar-free), scallions, sea vegetables (kelp, dulse, nori, etc.)
- Snow peas, snap peas, sprouts
- Squash: zucchini, yellow, summer, spaghetti
- Tomatoes or mixed vegetable juice (low sodium)
- Water chestnuts: 5 whole

STARCHY/SWEET VEGETABLES: 1 serving

1 serving = approximately 45 calories
Serving size: 1/2 cup, or as indicated

- Beets, winter squash (acorn, butternut)
- Carrots:½ cup cooked or 2 medium raw or 12 baby carrots
- Sweet potatoes or yams: 1/2 medium
- Yukon gold, new, or red potato: 1/2 medium

FRUITS: 1–2 servings

1 serving = approximately 80 calories
Serving size as indicated

- Apple: 1 medium
- Apricots: 3 medium
- Berries: blackberries and blueberries, 1 cup
- Raspberries and strawberries: 1 1/2 cups
- Cantaloupe: 1/2 medium
- Cherries: 15

- Fresh figs: 2
- Grapefruit: 1 whole
- Grapes: 15
- Honeydew melon: 1/4 small
- Kiwi: 2 medium
- Mango: 1/2 medium
- Nectarines: 2 small
- Orange: 1 large
- Peaches: 2 small
- Pear: 1 small
- Plums: 2 small
- Persimmon or pomegranate: 1/2

GRAINS (gluten-free): 1 serving

1 serving = approximately 75–100 calories

Serving Size: 1/2 cup cooked, or as indicated

- Basmati or other brown rice, wild rice
- Buckwheat
- Millet
- Quinoa

HEALTHY FATS: 4–5 servings

1 serving = approximately 40 calories

Serving size: 1 teaspoon, or as indicated

Oils should be cold pressed

Plant Oils (salads, veggies, etc.)

- Avocado (fruit): 1/8
- Coconut milk (canned), light: 3 tablespoons
- Coconut milk (canned), regular: 1 1⁄2 tablespoons
- Flaxseed oil (refrigerate)
- Olives: 8–10 medium
- Olive oil, extra virgin (preferable)
- Sesame oil

Cooking Oils

- Olive oil, avocado oil
- Coconut oil
- Ghee (clarified butter) • Grapeseed oil

CONDIMENTS

Servings per day: As much or as little as you desire

- Unsweetened tomato sauce or salsa
- Mustard
- Fresh or dried herbs (any): basil, sage, rosemary, mint, parsley, etc.
- Fresh or dried spices (any): curry, paprika, chili powder, etc.

BEVERAGES

Up to 8 glasses, 8 ounces each

- Water (ideally filtered)
- Mineral water (still or carbonated)
- Rooibos, tulsi tea (unsweetened)
- Non-caffeinated herbal teas (mint, chamomile, hibiscus, etc.)

RADIANT TIP

HORMONE BALANCING DIET

- Eat lots of fresh fruits and vegetables.
- Consume adequate protein.
- Enjoy moderate amounts of healthy fats.
- Eat plenty of fiber.
- Drink lots of fresh water or herbal tea.

WHAT ABOUT WINE?

Most women I meet love wine. Paired with the right healthy meal combination, wine can complement a health plan and even offer some health benefits. Red wine contains resveratrol, which has been linked with longevity. A nice glass of wine can help you relax into the joy of life, although it's good to remember that wine adds to your carbs, so you want to look at the total sugar you're bringing into your body each day. On the days you're drinking wine, consider having less fruit or starchy vegetables. Exercise and hydrate to balance.

And how are you using the wine? Is it something to enhance your meal and help you relax? Or are you using it to cover up emotions and numb out the things you don't want to deal with? Has it become a habit?

By pausing and asking these questions, we regain control and allow ourselves pleasure. When choosing wine, choose organic, sulfite-free, biodynamic wines for ideal health and wellness.

Salud!

COFFEE

Who doesn't love the rich aroma and taste of coffee in the morning to wake up our brains and get into the flow of our day? (I DO, I DO!) I'm here to say, give your coffee an upgrade. Coffee is a highly sprayed crop. Buy organic when possible. Who wants to be digesting extra toxins and pesticides? (I sure don't!) You want the highest-grade coffee you can find. And if you're adding creamer or milk, consider swapping out the popular chemical-laden brands for a healthier alternative like unsweetened coconut, soy, or other plant-based milk. Additionally, there are lots of exciting new plant-based coffee creamer combos available. Look for them in the refrigerator section at your local market or health food store.

Coffee has some health benefits. As mentioned in Gut 101, coffee contains healthy acids like chlorogenic acid, polyphenols, and antioxidant compounds, which have prebiotic properties. In Chinese medicine coffee is used for medicinal purposes to help activate metbolism and support proper elimination. Coffee also boosts dopamine, that feel-good hormone we love.

When consuming coffee, ask yourself how much you are having. Is it two cups or ten? (I once had a client who was drinking nine cups of coffee a day just to stay afloat and energetic. She dropped that habit to two cups after a 21-day cleanse and new food plan.)

Be aware, too, that coffee has a 1.5 to 9.5 hour half-life, with the average being about 5-6 hours.

The caffeine can impede your sleep if you're sensitive (even decaf, which has a small amount of caffeine). I recommend drinking coffee in the morning before noon, and preferably before 10 a.m. Put it in your favorite mug and sip, savor, and enjoy.

LET'S TALK ABOUT HYDRATION. ARE YOU DRINKING ENOUGH WATER?

We've heard it over and over again: "Drink more water."

But the truth is, water is the most essential ingredient for good health. You could potentially change the trajectory of your aging process just by drinking more water and staying hydrated. Honesty, it's one of the best anti-aging potions on the planet.

Our bodies are 70 percent water. (check) Every cell in our body needs water to function. (check) Cells have their own detoxification system, so they're always releasing toxins and chemicals. And water helps flush out waste from daily cellular function.

Water is also important for brain health, so if you're not thinking clearly, drink water.

(Think of a plant that lacks water. It wilts! Same goes for YOU.) The body also gets dehydrated as you're sleeping. It repairs itself while you sleep, so you wake up in a more acidic state. A way to regain balance is to drink a glass of water or two upon awakening.

Water supports:

1. A better mood
2. More energy
3. Less fatigue
4. Better digestion/regularity
5. Sharper focus/better concentration
6. Lubricated tissues and joints
7. Fewer sugar cravings
8. Weight loss/better metabolism
9. Clear, radiant skin
10. Improved health and overall well-being

RADIANT TIP

BENEFITS OF WATER

1. Dissolves nutrients so that they are more easily absorbed in the digestive tract.
2. Transports nutrients to cells and tissues.
3. Carries wastes and materials from cells to kidneys for filtration and elimination.
4. Absorbs and transports heat; boosts metabolism.
5. Supports glowing, dewy skin.

HOW MUCH WATER SHOULD I DRINK?

No single formula fits everyone. The National Academy of Sciences, Engineering and Medicine determined that an average daily fluid intake for women is 11.5 cups. This recommendation includes water, other beverages, and food. Regarding water: A good rule of thumb is to divide your body weight in half and drink that in ounces. So, if you weigh 120 pounds, you'd want to consider drinking 60 ounces (or 6–7 cups) of water a day. Herbal teas count as well. If exercising and sweating, you will want to replenish the water in your body. If you're thirsty, then you're already dehydrated. You want to catch that before it happens.

NOTE: A healthy diet full of lots of juicy fruits and vegetables contributes to a body that is hydrated.

Some of us have trouble drinking plain water, so do whatever you need to make water palatable. A squeeze of lemon adds brightness but also alkalizes water. Make your own spa water with cucumbers and herbs or berries and mint.

RADIANT TIP

BOOKEND YOUR DAY WITH WATER

Start your day with water. If you get in one to two cups right away in the morning, then you're already well on your way to proper hydration—especially before your coffee. Before you dehydrate, hydrate. The purer the water, the better. In the evening, have another cup or two of water or herbal tea.

Okay, let's take what we've learned. I'll share a few more tips, and set you up for a perfect day of wellness.

Chapter 7

RADIANT DAY:
A DAY OF WELLNESS

The simple things we do each day
create the joy and happiness we crave.

– D R .   D E A N   O R N I S H

We live in a wonderful time where modern technology allows us to fly across the country on airplanes and text our loved ones midair. We find old friends on Facebook and direct message new friends on Instagram. But sometimes these opportunities can take us away from the present moment and the simplicity of our lives.

Just for today, let's keep things simple. Let's start by connecting to our breath. To know we are alive and that we can make small incremental changes, step by step, moment by moment.

Just for today, let's savor something nourishing: a fresh vegetable, succulent fruit, or hydrating glass of water. Nutrition can be fun and playful. It doesn't have to mean eating a complex gourmet meal or implementing a complete change to our lifestyle.

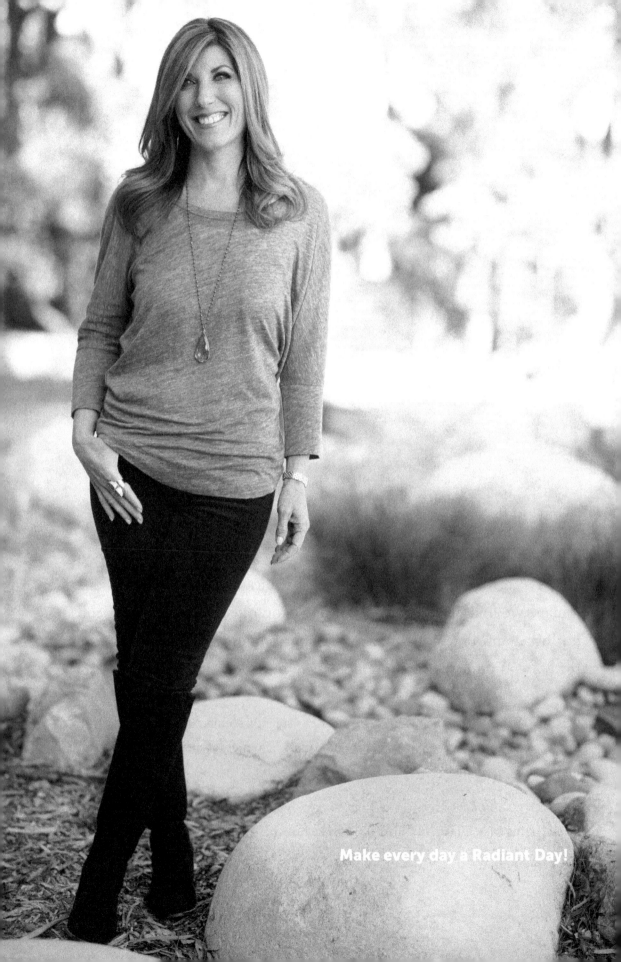

Make every day a Radiant Day!

At first, new habits and new beginnings can seem overwhelming or foreign. Remember your first day of high school, how different it seemed and how you wondered whether you would ever find all your classrooms? Over time, you figured out just where those classrooms were and high school became a comfortable part of your routine. Or remember when you first tried to ride a bike without training wheels? Then one day you got on and went confidently zooming down the street!

Anything new can be overwhelming or uncomfortable. When we embark on new lifestyle habits and move out of our comfort zone, *we discover where the magic happens!*

So, expect to be uncomfortable and know that you are moving toward your greater desires and goals.

Just for today, be gentle with yourself. Give your new routine and your new habits time to unfold. Be forgiving of yourself if you fall down or take a step off the path. And if you happen to get lost in your old ways, stand up, love yourself, and gently step back on the road.

Just for today, let's sprinkle our morning, noon, and evening with loving kindness. Loving kindness means loving ourselves and others despite our mistakes and struggles, and that means theirs too. Remember, we are human. We make mistakes and that's how we learn and grow.

RADIANT TIP

YOU'RE WORTH IT!

You're worth your own love and self-care. Wellness is not about the number on the scale. Wellness is not about fitting into our skinny jeans (even though that is fun and very rewarding). Wellness is about our mental, physical, emotional, and spiritual well-being coming together in peace and harmony.

HOW TO DESIGN A DAY OF HEALTH

The secret to creating a day of health is to make yourself a priority and put simple daily practices and routines in place that support well-being.

SIMPLE, CLEAN, AND CONSISTENT ROUTINES

Each day when we rise, we want to build a strong foundation and create a path for radiant health. The pull of the day can be so strong, especially if you're a doer. Before you pick up your phone to read through emails and the news or scroll through Instagram, give yourself some me time. If you have kids or need to care for family members, consider getting up earlier to carve out some time for YOU. Your morning me time can be tailored to your personal liking. There is no perfect way to do it. My top recommendations include:

- A short meditation, visualization, reflection, or setting an intention for the day
- A relaxing cup of organic coffee, herbal tea, or matcha latte
- Reading for ten minutes from an inspirational book
- Walking your dog (This can be done as a walking meditation too.)
- Morning movement/exercise. Morning is a great time to move. It will set you up with energy and mood-boosting hormones all day long.

You can't pour from an empty cup. Take care of yourself first.

Think of self-care as a habit that pays off in spades. Personally, I wake up early most every day to meditate, write, and visualize what I want for the day. I enjoy my morning coffee in peace and use the quiet time to be in creative thought. I bring my own snacks when I travel and am intentional about the restaurants I frequent and the products I purchase. I pause to take breath breaks throughout the day and put on my favorite essential oils to protect my energy and uplift my mood, especially if I'm entering into a tough conversation or a crowded space or freeway. When you invest in your self-care, you invest in your longer-term health.

BUILD HABITS THAT ARE ENJOYABLE AND SUSTAINABLE

EAT BASED ON THE BLOOD-SUGAR BALANCING PROPERTIES OF FAT, FIBER, AND PROTEIN.

This way of eating keeps our blood sugar balanced and our bodies happy. It also helps us feel full, calm, and fueled. Build your plate with the healthy foods you like. Create a structure that *you* can stick with. When you understand the how and why of the habits you wish to change, you are so much more motivated to make healthy choices.

- Look at trends as tools. You can incorporate pieces. Avoid extremes.
- Pick something that is executable. Be consistent. Infuse discipline.
- If you know you won't have time for breakfast, blend your smoothie the night before, or make an extra one or two and freeze. Then grab and go.
- Eat to improve your health.
- Eat to achieve your goals.
- Focus on balanced and nutrient-dense meals.
- Mini milestones help keep you motivated and on track.

RADIANT TIP

HOW TO STAY IN BALANCE

Let go of the expectation that life should always look a certain way. Recognize that life is fluid and what we need one day may be completely different from what we need another day. Recognize that our future is created today. The only time we have is NOW. A big part of staying in balance is being present and recognizing when we're out of balance too.

RITUALS, ROUTINES, AND NON-NEGOTIABLES

WELLNESS FOR A GREAT DAY

- Morning me time
- Breakfast
- Lunch
- Snack
- Dinner
- Evening wind down

MORNING: ME TIME

MORNING PRACTICES

Here are some of my favorite healthy rituals and practices that I recommend to my clients. You can pick one, start there, stick with it, or add others that work for you one at a time.

- Drink a 6–8 ounce glass of lemon water.
- Take supplements that support your gut and/or skin and/or contain antioxidants.
- Have coffee or tea.
- Meditate, pray, or otherwise connecting with your inside (essential!).
- Set morning intentions or visualize what you want for the day.
- Read or listen to something inspirational for 10–20 minutes.
- Do breath work.
- Move, exercise, or walk the dog.
- Have a healthy breakfast built on fat, fiber and protein.

WHAT WOULD MARLYN DO?

MY DAILY RITUALS

Over the years, I've had a variety of clients tell me that when they're stuck on a food choice or deciding what to do, they ask themselves, "What would Marlyn do?" They also ask me how I go about my day. So, here's a sneak peak:

I wake up between 5 a.m. and 6 a.m., and start my day with a few basic high-quality supplements. I drink lemon water, organic coffee, and then a protein shake. (See list of choices in Chapter 10.) Once I've organized my day, I make room for an hour of exercise, which varies but can include walking, hiking, strength training class, or Cardio Barre. On most days, I start work at 9 a.m., though because I work from home, I often begin earlier, especially if I'm writing or creating a seminar or an online project. When I coach clients on the East Coast, whose timetable is three hours ahead of mine, I'm often ready at 7 or 8 a.m.

- Lemon water (super hydrating, alkalizing)
- Supplements (1 probiotic, 1 alpha-lipoic acid)
- Coffee (1 ½ cups, organic French roast with unsweetened soy milk, which I LOVE!)
- Meditation (ten minutes, sometimes more; this is life-changing)
- Read something inspirational for 10–20 minutes (plug into the positive)
- Write (this book!, a blog post, Instagram post, or journal entry)
- Some days, I intermittently fast before I work out. Other days, I might have 1–2 teaspoons of almond butter to keep my blood sugar stable.
- Work out/Barre class/hike (I love to be in nature)
- On the mornings I work out, I have a shake or light breakfast afterward.
- Meet with a client, work on a project, plan a live event, or get ready for talk

For lunch, I like to include lots of colorful veggies and simple proteins. Some days I'll toss together a variety of leafy greens (I especially love endive!) and any other vegetables in my fridge to make a big beautiful colorful rainbow salad with avocado, extra virgin olive oil (I LOVE the really good pure varieties from Italy, which are my liquid gold), fresh lemon juice, and pink salt. If I'm craving a bit of fish, I'll pop open a tin of wild sardines to top off the salad. I enjoy sardines that are boneless/skinless and packed in olive oil from Morocco, which have no fishy taste and are great brain food.

Other days, I find myself enjoying leftovers from the neighborhood healthy Indian takeout I ordered the night before (see my suggestions in Chapter 11) or the Baked Salmon (recipe in Capter 10) I made with roasted sweet potatoes (recipe in Capter 10) or quinoa and broccoli (recipe in Capter 10). My general rule of thumb is to feed my body good, healthy food and listen for the cues of what I may be craving. Dinner is an array of roasted veggies, sweet potatoes, and/or quinoa (if I didn't have it at lunch) and salad or stews, depending on the season and my activity level that day. My main intention each day when choosing meals or snacks is to listen to my body and aim to give it what it needs to feel great.

RADIANT TIP

WHAT YOU EAT +
HOW YOU LOOK AND FEEL

I believe the connection between what we eat and the way we look and feel is extraordinarily powerful. As I've shared throughout these pages, in my experience food has the power to regenerate, heal, ignite, and energize us. I also believe food has the power to change our moods on a dime and derail our best intentions, be the catalyst for fights and upsets in relationships, and ruin our sleep and relaxation. It's a huge factor in our mental and emotional well-being and has much to do with the energy we have during the day and the things we get done in this lifetime. With every choice I make, I ask myself, "How is this food going to make me feel?" and, "What effect is this food going to have on my health?" Then I choose accordingly. Every day is an adventure, and honestly, choosing foods that are delicious and good for my body contributes to my self-esteem and self-confidence.

HERE'S A FEW IDEAS FOR A RADIANT DAY OF EATING:

SAMPLE DAY 1

Breakfast: Smoothie, oatmeal, or muesli bowl (recipe in Capter 10)

Lunch: Sliced pear with small handful of walnuts (8)

Snack: 5–8 flax crackers with ¼ mashed avocado and sea salt

Dinner: Roasted wild salmon with broccoli rabe and steamed brown rice

SAMPLE DAY 2

Breakfast: Smoothie or veggie omelette

Lunch: Lettuce wraps with grilled shrimp and avocado

Snack: ¼ cup of hummus with cucumber spears

Dinner: Organic roast chicken with grilled vegetables and quinoa

SAMPLE DAY 3

Breakfast: Smoothie or warming grain-free bowl

Lunch: Farmer's market veggie salad with grilled salmon

Snack: Brenda's famous guacamole with baby carrots (recipe, Chapter 10)

Dinner: Lentil stew with roasted sweet potatoes and veggies

RADIANT TIP

HIGH-POWERED IMMUNE-BOOSTING EATING

We're in the midst of a changing world. The state of our health and the efficiency of our immune systems has become more important than ever. Eating immune-boosting foods and drinking immune-boosting teas and tonics is a fantastic way to care for ourselves. Consider adding in these foods, drinks, and lifestyle rituals for a day of immunity-boosting wellness.

- ½ cup of berries
- ½ tsp. rosemary + ½ tsp. turmeric (add to stews or salads or rub on chicken)
- 1 medium clove garlic, roasted or raw (raw garlic contains higher amounts of allicin, which supports immunity)
- 2 cups of dark leafy veggies
- 2 cups of cruciferous veggies: broccoli, cabbage, cauliflower, Brussels sprouts, bok choy, arugula, kale, watercress, rutabaga, kohlrabi, radish, turnip
- 3 cups of low-glycemic colorful veggies

- Don't eat between 7 p.m. and 7 a.m.
- Stay hydrated
- Choose organic at least half the time
- Include healthy oils
- Avoid dairy

Immunity Boost Bonus:
- 1–2 cups of green tea (If sensitive to caffeine, have tea earlier in the day)
- 1–2 cups of oolong tea (If sensitive to caffeine, have tea earlier in the day)

BUILDING HEALTH
IS A STEP-BY-STEP APPROACH

Start with one baby step at a time, one action step at a time, one teaspoon of change at a time. Toss out one chemical-laden food from your pantry. Add in one new green vegetable. Swap up your food choices from processed to fresh. Over time, all those baby steps turn into a glorious journey.

WHAT THE HECK CAN I DO WITH AN AVOCADO?

Amazing, voluptuous avocados are loaded with healthy fats (which keep the top layer of our skin moist and beautiful), oleic acid (which helps lower cholesterol), and lots of fiber (keeping us satiated and fuller longer). They also help us moderate cortisol, the stress hormone. Add some to your smoothie or mash on gluten-free toast. Blend some up in the blender with raw cacao and almond milk for a chocolate dairy-free pudding treat. Make a homemade guacamole or just a plain ol' avocado mash with sea salt and cayenne pepper. Cut up some jicama or Persian cucumbers for a great afternoon snack. The possibilities are endless.

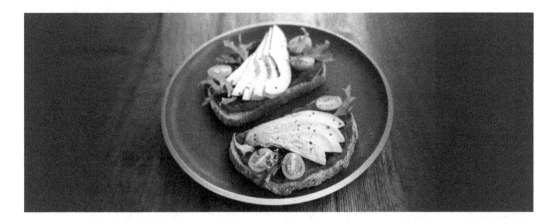

MIDDAY/AFTERNOON

Lunch: Healthy meal, salad, or soup with protein. Think fat, fiber, and protein.

Afternoon snack: Many of us tend to have a blood sugar dip around 3 or 4 p.m.

That's the time you see the lines at Starbucks get longer. Before that energy dip happens, catch it with a fat, fiber, and protein-based snack. It could be as simple as a handful of pumpkin seeds.

Breath break: Instead of an afternoon coffee break, take a breath break. Afternoon is a great time to pause and take a few conscious, deep, mindful breaths. The oxygen will fuel your body and brain and help bring you back to the present moment.

Essential oils: Along with a good balanced snack, essential oils are a great way to keep your vibe high throughout the day. I'm usually applying my balance grounded oil or adaptive calm oil (both by doTERRA). I love the way they enhance my mood and ground my mind back down into my body.

Get out in nature: To avoid the afternoon slump, get out and take a walk— even if it's a walk around the block to look at the flowers and the trees. This is great if you've been in the house or office all day or are going through a stressful moment. Nature is uplifting. Take a moment to look at the blue sky, feel the wind on your skin, and smell the air. Most of the time, we live in our heads and forget to look around and notice the beauty around us.

RADIANT TIP

TAKE A TEA BREAK

Tea breaks are the best. Spend tea time with your beloved BFF, colleague, or your glorious SELF.

Teas in general are loaded with healing properties. Many teas, like green, white, chai, chamomile, and bergamot, are naturally abundant with antioxidants and polyphenols that help lower inflammation in the body and balance hormones. Ginger and mint are great for digestion. Chamomile and rooibos are super to support a good night's sleep. Most every night I make myself a cup of tea. My favorite is rooibos or chamomile. The tea is calming and soothing and reminds me to slow down. It also reminds me that it is nighttime and it lets my body know it's time for bed. It's a great ritual to implement and also a way to calm the body and mind down at the end of the day.

DINNER

Dinner: Think fat, fiber, and protein. Check out the recipes in the recipe section. Depending on your activity for the day, you might consider having a small amount of slow carbs (½ cup or ½ potato). Quinoa, sweet potatoes, and brown rice are especially nice for many in the evening, as they have high levels of sleep-promoting complex carbohydrates and naturally calming magnesium, which may help you relax before bedtime.

Intermittent Fasting: If you want to lose weight or help heal your blood sugar or insulin resistance, consider finishing dinner by 7 or 8 p.m. and call it a day for your food consumption.

BEDTIME: EVENING WIND DOWN

Let's face it: if you're not getting good quality sleep, you're going to suffer. Sleep is one of the most important things contributing to our optimal health and well-being. Without good quality, deep, restful sleep, we tend to crave more carbs, wrestle with unpleasant moods, and sacrifice our best energy for the things we love. Research shows immunity is higher with good sleep, and with sleep deprivation we are more susceptible to infectious agents. Consider getting a minimum of 6–8 hours of restful sleep each night for maximum rejuvenation and regeneration. Give yourself the gift of sleep.

TOP TIPS FOR A GREAT NIGHT'S SLEEP

To promote restful restorative sleep, try the following routine.
- Eat a relatively light dinner. Stop eating around 7 or 8 p.m.
- Take a leisurely stroll after dinner.
- Take a bath before bed. Create a spa-like experience.
- Diffuse relaxing aromas in your bedroom. Listen to soothing music.
- Drink a cup of warm relaxing herbal tea.
- Read inspirational or spiritual literature for a few minutes before bed.
- Sleep in a dark bedroom. Use black-out shades, cover any dim lights on clocks, computers, televisions, etc.

- Once in bed, close your eyes and simply feel your body—this means focus on your body and wherever you notice tension, consciously relax that area.

3 THINGS I PERSONALLY LOVE AND USE FOR BETTER SLEEP

Magnesium: Most of us are deficient in magnesium. This essential mineral is needed for over 300 metabolic processes in the body—including heart health, blood sugar regulation and bone health. Magnesium is less abundant in our soils than it was years ago. If you have trouble sleeping, you might consider adding a magnesium supplement to your nightly routine. I personally take a buffered magnesium glycinate formula each night before bed. This high-performance chelated product helps to calm the nervous system and supports a more relaxing night's rest.

Cortisol Manager: If you've got stress, chances are you've got high amounts of cortisol, too! Cortisol does have some positive attributes and is needed by the body, although high amounts circulating over time can lead to inflammation, unwanted weight gain, and many sleepless nights. Cortisol Manager by Integrative Therapeutics is a formula I personally love and recommend to my clients for a better night's sleep. This natural healing supplement is made from ashwagandha, phosphatidylserine, L-theanine, and calming flower essences like magnolia. It's also non-addictive.

Serenity Essential Oil by doTERRA: This is an amazing, beautifully scented essential oil made by my favorite essential oil company, doTERRA. Serenity is a blend of lavender, chamomile, and vanilla designed to relax and heal the body and mind. For a deeper, more restorative sleep, consider putting 1–3 drops on each foot before bed. Rub in and voila, you are gently transported into deep relaxation and bliss. Great for kids and teens, too.

As you lay your head on your pillow, take a few deep breaths and focus on all the beauty and blessings in your life. Consider doing a brain dump—where you literally dump all that crazy stuff floating around in your head on a piece of paper. This allows the mind to rest in a more peaceful, relaxing manner.

STRESS

Stress often leads to physical and psychological changes within the body that can have long-lasting side effects. Ongoing stress sets off a series of hormonal reactions that can contribute to anxiety, tension, sleepless nights, hormonal imbalances, and chronic disease. Stress is one of the biggest driving factors contributing to poor health and weight gain. It can affect the body in ways that are difficult to see from the outside. It can lead to emotional eating, high blood pressure, heartburn, thyroid imbalance, and more.

RADIANT TIP

STRESS SOOTHERS

Use essential oils like lavender, citrus, and chamomile.

Go outside and take a walk. Listen to relaxing music. Light a candle.

Take stretch breaks. If you're working at a desk, get up and take a break every ninety minutes.

Have some soothing tea, like rooibos, chamomile, or holy basil.

RADIANT TIP

THE WELL-NOURISHED HOME

As we continue to nurture our minds, bodies and spirit, we also want to nurture our precious living spaces. Think of your home as your second skin. You want to keep the good energy flowing and the harmful elements out. With a fresh perspective, ask yourself, "How does my home make me feel?" What brings my loved ones and me joy? What no longer inspires or energizes me? Trust your senses – sight, sound, touch, and smell. Fill your home with elements that uplift your optimal health and wellbeing. Simple treats like fresh flowers, a candle made with essential oils, a cozy pillow sewn with natural fibers.

DIANA'S WELLNESS JOURNEY UPDATE

Nine-Pound Weight Loss

We are three months into Diana's wellness journey and she has lost nine pounds. She has also become a certified mediator, which was one of her goals.

I asked Diana to reflect on all the things she's been doing to support her success. Here's what she shared: "I've taken the positive energy and support from our coaching sessions and created my own formula for a day of wellness. This gives me structure, a blueprint to follow, and peace of mind. Personally, I THRIVE on structure!

"Also, you recommended that I chose a word as an overarching theme for my wellness journey. I chose the word ALIGN, and I find myself using it a lot. Alignment has become my compass, my truth, my inner guide, especially when I'm faced with making a decision around food or lifestyle habits. I often ask myself, are the foods I'm eating, choices I'm making, and my daily habits in ALIGNMENT with my wellness goals? Are negative thought patterns, old stories, black-and-white thinking in alignment with my greater joy and happiness?

"My intention each day is to stay in alignment with my bigger picture goals."

In addition to making more conscious food choices, Diana focused her attention on creating new, healthier habits. As a way to ground Diana in her own success and help her celebrate positive changes, I asked her to name the healthy habits she has been practicing so she would get VERY CLEAR on what has been supporting her.

Below are her reflections.

"Healthy habits that give consistent structure to my day:

1. **Each night before bed I journal.** I write down at least three things I'm grateful for, without fail. Sometimes it's three words. Other times, it's three sentences (or more!).

2. **Fun things I did today.** I also journal about the fun things I do. Again, sometimes it's just a few words, other times it's a couple of sentences or a short paragraph. It reminds me to have fun and enjoy my life.

3. **Habit tracker:** A guidebook that helps me measure whether I'm building good habits. This gives me structure and helps me stick with my routine. I like the book *Clear Habit Tracker* by James Clear. It's simple, clear, and easy to use.

4. **What I wore.** I do this for the fun of it. I write in my journal what I wore that day. It gives me insight into how I was feeling.

5. **Atomic Habits.** This book by James Clear is phenomenal, and reading it along with my biweekly nutrition coaching sessions has helped me shift my mindset. It gave me an understanding of how habits form and what it takes to truly change them. **Hint:** Focus on what you want to achieve and take the first step toward it. And when you're comfortable with the first step, take the second.

6. **Meditating for three minutes.** I set a timer and meditate every night without fail. Three minutes makes it doable. This habit has been life-changing. I've become calmer and more aware during the day. And, on top of that, I'm so proud of myself for STICKING WITH IT!

7. **Vary exercise.** I love to mix it up! I keep it fun. Biking, weights, Pilates, etc.

8. **Gave up "all or nothing" thinking.** I now live in the Gray Zone. I've been an "all or nothing" thinker my whole life. I love this new way of being.

9. **Let go of "should not."** I let go of harsh judgment and became more open-minded.

10. **ACE: Add in, Crowd out, Elevate up!** I adopted this practice and LOVE IT! It's SO helpful and truly supports my daily food choices. It's been a HUGE part of my mindset shift. For example, if I want some chocolate (which I love!), I elevate up and choose the highest quality brand, avoiding the highly processed sugars and chemicals. I find I eat less and enjoy my treat more.

11. **STICK-TO-ITIVENESS attitude!** On occasion I run into resistance, like when the scale won't move, or when I'd much rather stay home and sip my matcha tea latte rather than hit the gym. Then I remember the word STICK-TO-ITIVENESS, and poof! It pulls me forward and back in alignment. I love this word and newfound mindset."

Diana completes her wellness journey in Chapter 11 and shares her best tips for staying committed, calm, and on track every day.

HONOR ALL THE PARTS

In 2014, I first learned about the power of honoring all our parts from Dr. David Allen, and I have used it ever since in my personal life and in my coaching practice. It's especially eye-opening and helpful when applied to relationships. The truth is, we all have different parts that make up who we are. If we hide, judge, squash, or feel ashamed about some of our parts, it diminishes who we truly are on the inside. Our relationships to ourselves and each other (self-love and romantic love) will be as healthy and fulfilling to the degree we feel comfortable bringing in all our parts. In other words, the degree to which we are comfortable sharing all our parts is the degree to which we will experience fulfilling relationships and be appreciated for who we truly are.

WELCOME ALL THE PARTS OF OUR PRECIOUS SELVES

- We are all made up of parts.

- We all have parts that want to be healthy.
- Parts that don't care very much.
- Parts that want to be in relationships.
- Parts that want to be on our own.
- Parts that want to be happy.
- Parts that are more serious.
- Parts that want to exercise.
- Parts that want to sit and relax.

We honor and welcome all of the parts that make us whole. We even welcome our inner critic and forgive ourselves. Let's take an example. For many, there's a part who loves sugar. There's nothing inherently wrong with sugar or sweets of any kind. But if we eat too many cookies, donuts, and Snickers bars, the part of us who wants to be healthy and fit may suffer. As we build our sense of self, we become aware of these different parts, how they are sometimes at odds with one another. Over time, we want to develop acceptance of those parts and the discipline to avoid the pitfalls they may lead us into. In other words, we become more human. From our deepest humanity, we can actualize our deepest authenticity knowing that the path of authenticity is the most powerful path of all. And yes, it's okay to love a delicious cookie every now and then.

HOW TO RECLAIM YOUR PERSONAL POWER

MEETING UP AGAIN WITH YOUR WISEST, WILDEST HEART.

As part of your healing journey you must reclaim your power and dignity. This goes above and beyond food. It goes straight to the places where we have given away our power over a lifetime. When we hit the mid-stage and scan back over our lives, most of us will find a moment (or two, or three, or more) where we faced trauma, upset, abuse, bullying, or injustice.

Sometimes it happened because we were young and didn't have the power, wisdom, or know-how to use our voice.

Sometimes it happened because we were unaware that another whom we trusted acted without our knowledge or permission and that act led to unfortunate circumstances or a change in the way we thought our life would unfold.

And sometimes, it happened because we were naive and we let ourselves get talked into something that was not in our best interest.

When we face these moments in our lives, many of us may turn to food or alcohol as a way to cope, to numb out, or to feel better. And yes, this may be helpful and sometimes exactly what is needed in a stressful moment. But after a while, what begins as a way to comfort ourselves may turn into a self-destructive act, which can cause more harm than good (like becoming vulnerable to type 2 diabetes from eating too much sugar and high-carb food).

I want you to know that it is possible to reclaim your power. You can reclaim the parts of yourself you gave away. The following is a brief overview of how I approach reclaiming power with my clients, and how I've helped heal myself along the way, as well.

OKAY, READY? START NOW.

Sit in a quiet, comfortable place where your body and mind can relax. Close your eyes. Breathe deeply in and out of your nose. Breathe in compassion and breathe out love toward yourself. Bring your breath to your heart. Breathe in kindness and compassion toward yourself. You truly are your body's best friend.

Now, gently look for a moment where your dignity and power were stripped from you. It could be with friends, partners, parents, grandparents, teachers, relatives, siblings, neighbors, bosses, or a person on the subway.

Once you have a picture of a specific moment, gently reimagine what happened and reply to the person who hurt you. Let them know how you were blindsided or unable to defend yourself. Be aware of any judgment you have of yourself. Know that you did what you knew best at the time and you most likely operated from a place of survival.

Now, with that part of yourself in your mind, love yourself up. Give yourself the power to say or do what you really wanted to do or say, as if you would not suffer ANY consequences for doing it or saying it. Give yourself a voice. Let yourself say all the things that you wish you had said back then. You can do this silently or out loud. You could write it down as well.

And know this. You are on the path to reclaim your power and dignity. You are on the path to healing.

When I work with clients, if they're willing, I help them with this exercise. Because even if we could not do anything then, we *can* do something *now*. And this is the part where you get to mother yourself. You get to love up all the parts of you that you wish you could have changed. And you get to appreciate and love up all the lessons too, because they have brought you forward to be the amazing person you are today.

You can begin to look at your relationship with food in a new way. To see if food or alcohol was your coping mechanism and if you are still immersed in those old habits. It's never too late to change. It's never too late to re-create your relationship with yourself and your life.

Every moment is an opportunity for a new beginning. Healing starts with you. I'm here cheering you on every step of the way.

THOUGHTS ON EATING, AGING, AND LIVING STRONG:

1. Understand the connection between what you eat and how you feel.
2. Notice what's going on with your body as you age.
   Feed it what it needs to thrive.
3. Chuck standard beliefs about aging. Feel better as you age.
4. Explore practices to feel your best: me time, meditation, nature walks, etc.
5. We are all unique and we need different things to feel great.
6. Figure out the formula for your own well-being.
7. Eat food that supports your optimal health.
8. Small changes go a long way. No matter what age you are, you can change.
9. Nourishing yourself with good food is not about being perfect.
10. You can be a gourmet cook or an assembler. Just get back into the kitchen.
11. Choose and eat ingredients that help you improve with time.
12. The brain is 60 percent fat. Feed it good fats.

We've got our day down. We're reclaiming our power. We've learned new ways to care for ourselves. **Now, let's go shopping!**

Chapter 8

THE SHOPPING LIST

*The food you eat can either be the safest
and most powerful form of medicine
or the slowest form of poison.*

– ANN WIGMORE

HEALTHY ESSENTIALS
SHOPPING LIST

One of the best gifts you can give yourself and your family is to stock your kitchen or office fridge with foods full of nourishment and life force. In Sanskrit, life force is known as *prana*, which means breath or primary energy. In Chinese, it's known as *chi*. Foods full of natural life force and healthy, pleasurable ingredients lead to creating mindful meals that satisfy more than just hunger—they also lead to a body full of vitality and a mind that is focused, clear, and alive.

When I work with a client, we begin with a pantry purge. Becoming aware of the kinds of foods we buy and consume is a huge step toward stress-free, healthy, energizing meals.

In your kitchen, I suggest you make your pantry purge into a game. Become a food sleuth. Take a moment and look around your kitchen and cupboards for chemical-laden foods and drinks. Be on further lookout for food additives, preservatives, hidden refined sugars, MSG, and added sodium. Review anything that is highly processed, packaged, canned, boxed, and baked. Read labels.

After you've gone through your pantry and purged, we're ready to fill up our shelves with lots of nutrient-dense, high-quality food, drinks, spices, herbs, condiments, and oils.

Let's make your kitchen a playful, color-filled healthy culinary space.

YOUR HEALTHY KITCHEN

FILL YOUR FRIDGE

A few things to consider: Alliums (garlic, onions, shallots): If you use them quickly (within a month), you can keep alliums in a drawer in your fridge. For longer periods, store them in the bottom pantry drawer in paper bags that have been punched with holes. For use within a week, hanging baskets are nice.

- Almond milk: homemade or store-bought with minimal ingredients
- Beets: Consider purchasing them precooked.
- Brassicas: Broccoli, Brussels sprouts, cabbage, cauliflower
- Carrots
- Celery
- Citrus fruits (lemons, limes, oranges, grapefruits)
- Endive
- Herbs (parsley, mint, basil, rosemary, cilantro, thyme)
- Kefir
- Leafy greens and lettuce (kale, arugula, romaine, spinach, radicchio)
- Root vegetables
- Tofu (soft, medium, or firm varieties): Opt for organic with minimal ingredients.

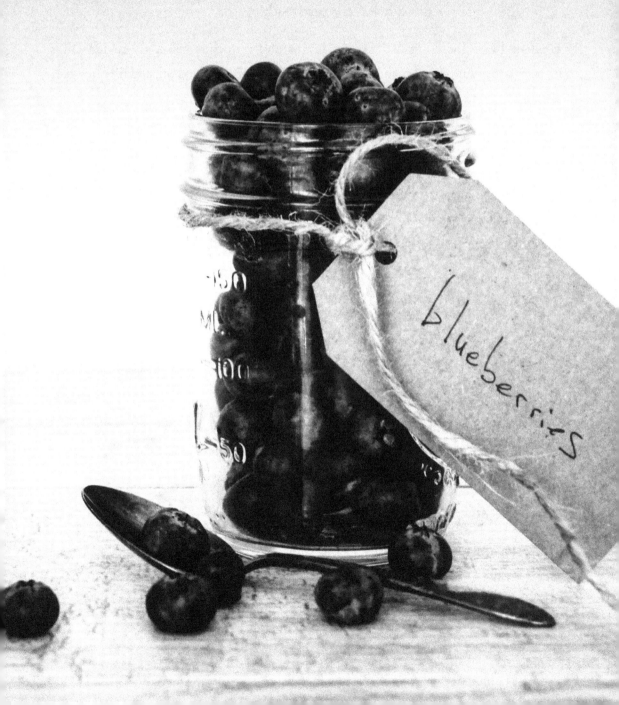

You are what you eat...
so eat well!

Protein

- Fish (wild): Seafood like shrimp, scallops, and crab are great choices too.
- Chicken (free range or organic): On occasion, I like to pick up a rotisserie-cooked chicken from my local market. Read the ingredients and look for simple things like organic chicken, sea salt. Avoid fillers, sodium nitrates, and other additives.
- Eggs (free range, organic, omega 3)
- Beef (grass-fed and organic, when possible)

Healthy Fats: These are fuel for our brains and mitochondria and provide anti-inflammatory support. Avocados, coconut oil, olive oil, flaxseed oil, and oily fish like salmon.

ON THE COUNTERTOP

Your countertop is a good place to display some of your favorite fruits and vegetables. Arrange them in pretty bowls or on a favorite plate. You're more likely to reach for the luscious treats in front of you than those hiding in the back of the fridge. Have fun with:

- Avocados
- Citrus: lemons, oranges, grapefruits, limes
- Fruit: seasonal fruits, bananas, apples, pears, peaches, etc.

WELLNESS PANTRY STAPLES

Some of my favorites:
- Beans (canned, BPA-free): black, chickpeas, pinto, kidney
- Coconut aminos: a gluten-free alternative to soy sauce
- Coconut milk (cartons and cans, BPA and additive-free
- Coconut oil (extra virgin, organic)
- Coffee (organic)
- Dijon mustard
- Gluten-free flours: almond, coconut, garbanzo bean
- Lentils: red, brown, yellow

- Rice: brown, wild, jasmine
- Olive oil (extra virgin) Oils: avocado, grape seed, walnut, sesame, and other nut and seed varieties
- Quinoa: yellow, sprouted, and/or multi-colored
- Nuts and seeds: almonds, walnuts, Brazil nuts, cashews, sunflower, pumpkin
- Chia seeds (organic)
- Flaxseeds (organic)
- Sardines (wild-caught boneless/skinless varieties packed in olive oil)
- Seaweed (sheets, shaker bottles)
- Spices: cinnamon, curry, ginger, nutmeg, oregano, red pepper flakes, blends
- Sweeteners: 100% maple syrup, honey (raw, manuka), lucama, monk fruit, coconut sugar
- Tahini (made from 100% sesame seeds)
- Tamari
- Vanilla bean powder
- Vinegars: balsamic, rice wine, apple cider

ADAPTOGENS: TRANSFORMATIONAL FOODS

For the alchemist in all of us, learning to upgrade our drinks, meals, and snacks with the ancient healing power of adaptogens can lead to a playful, creative, wellness boost. This list is a great place to start. Refer back to Chapter 5 for more on adaptogens.Maca

- Reishi
- Chaga
- Amla
- Pearl powder
- Ashwagandha
- Maca
- Cordyceps
- Shatavari
- Schisandra berry
- Mucuna pruriens

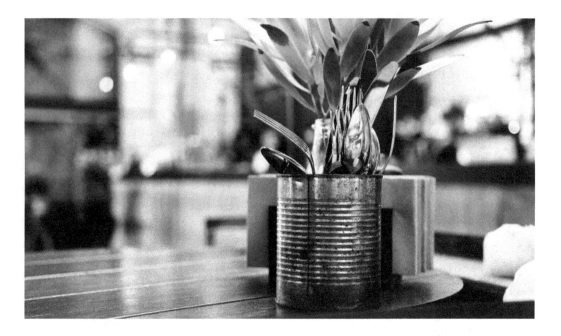

KITCHEN EQUIPMENT AND TOOLS

To create quick, easy-to-make meals, it's great to have a few go-to tools for cooking, prepping, and assembling.

- Blender: I love my Vitamix! Blendtec, NutriBullet, or other high-speed blenders work great too.
- Citrus press: This is wonderful for making homemade dressings or fresh lemon water.
- Colander/strainer: Use this to drain pasta, wash lettuce, or clean veggies.
- Cookware: Get ceramic, cast iron, or stoneware. It's fun to have a variety of sizes of pots and pans. I recommend: small 8", medium 10", and large 12–14". It's also useful to have various types: saucepans, stockpots, and sauté pans. Tip: Go for the best quality you can afford (even if that means investing in one good pan at a time).
- Cutting board: It's great having a small and medium cutting board to chop, cut, chiffonade, or slice vegetables, herbs, fruits, and meats.
- Measuring cups: Glass and metal cups are great. Be sure to get both dry and liquid measures.

- Microplane: You will love the simplicity of this gadget and the fresh taste of lemon, lime, grapefruit, or orange zest that it creates.
- Mixing bowls: Mix and match these for all your culinary needs.
- Nut milk bag: This is wonderful for making homemade nut milks.
- Peeler: Great for peeling and making zucchini/carrot/sweet potato ribbons.
- Potato masher: This is essential for homemade mashed potatoes or mashed cauliflower.
- Sheet pans: These are excellent for roasting veggies, nuts, or potatoes, and are also wonderful for baking up some gluten-free cookies and desserts.
- Spoons and spatulas: A variety of metal or bamboo spoons and spatulas make a wonderful addition to any culinary kitchen.
- Tongs
- Whisk

SUPPLEMENTS AND HOW TO USE THEM

A FEW THOUGHTS

HOW TO USE SUPPLEMENTS

Some of us need supplements. Others may not. When we get to midlife, there are a few supplements that can be quite supportive to our changing bodies—things like a good probiotic, vitamin D, magnesium, and perhaps curcumin or CoQ10. Supplements are not a perfect science. We use blood tests and our own body's innate wisdom and feedback to determine where to start.

In general, I recommend thinking of supplements as part of your diet. If you use supplements, consider looking for and purchasing the highest quality available. When choosing, look for high quality professional grade with no fillers or food additives and third-party tested. (GMP = good manufacturing practices.) NOTE: Consult with your physician or healthcare practitioner when choosing the best supplements for your health needs.

SUPPLEMENTS TO CONSIDER AFTER FIFTY

- Vitamin D
- Probiotic with high-quality ingredients
- Magnesium (mineral essential for production of energy)
- Multivitamin (look for high-quality ingredients including B vitamins for energy and cellular health)

MITOCHONDRIAL AND BLOOD SUGAR SUPPORT

- Alpha-lipoic acid
- Berberine
- Chromium
- Omega 3 fish oil
- Coenzyme Q10: This supports energy and protects the mitochondria. CoQ10 also supports biogenesis, the process of renewal and increase of mitochondrial cells.
- NAD+ is a key component involved in mitochondrial production of energy.
- NAD+ helps to make up several enzymes, including SIRT1 and SIRT3, which play key roles in healthy aging and weight management.

IMMUNITY AND RESPIRATORY SUPPORT

The following supplements may be very helpful in supporting the immune system as we age. I have listened to and read countless lectures and papers from highly accredited physicians on the front lines of research on disease and immunity. I especially enjoyed the presentation by Joel Evans, MD, who created and uploaded a clear and easily understandable online lecture about viruses and how to best support the body and immunity using food and high quality supplements. Below are a few supplements to consider for better immunity and respiratory support.

- Vitamin C (my favorite is buffered, as it is easier on the stomach)
- Zinc picolinate
- Vitamin D
- Resveratrol
- Quercetin
- Green tea

Note: Quantities of the above supplements will vary for each person, depending on age, health, and blood work.

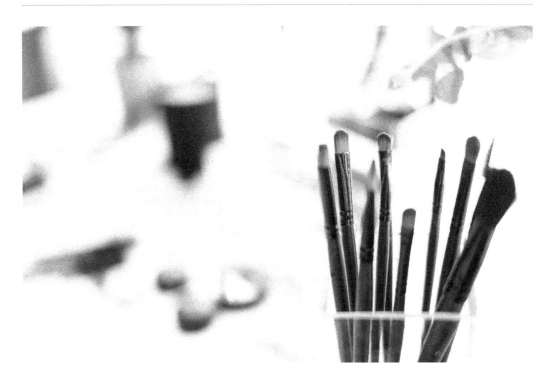

SKIN CARE

HOLISTIC, CLEAN, MINIMALISTIC APPROACH

Clean, green beauty is a growing phenomena. That's great news for all of us because what we put on our skin goes straight into our body. Be mindful when choosing cosmetics, skin care, and personal care products. Consider replacing one thing at a time as you use it up.

In Los Angeles, we have the Detox Market, which is a fantastic place to purchase and explore clean-label beauty products that are healthier for us and the environment. You can find the Detox Market online. Sephora is another establishment that has moved into the clean beauty space. Beautycounter is a woman-owned, rep-based company that has gorgeous products and extremely high standards around the ingredients they use.

SHOP MINDFULLY

Just like food, there is so much to discover here. Take your time and research products for your hair, skin, and nails and look for clean beauty markets in your area.

A FEW THINGS I LOVE:

- Epicurean: A brand I use for moisturizer and face wash. Rejuvenating.
- Coconut oil: This is a fabulous makeup remover, skin and hair nourisher, and lube!
- Dr. Bronner's: I love this body wash. It also has about ten other home uses.
- Dry brush or loofah: These are available at health markets and are great for lymphatic support.
- E.O.: They make bath and shower soaps, gels, oils, hand sanitizers, and lotions. Look for their products at local markets and online.
- Argan oil: This is a naturally occurring high-antioxidant plant oil from the argan nut and an excellent moisturizer for skin and hair. I get mine at Trader Joe's, which is 100% pure, organic, and very reasonably priced.

CONGRATULATIONS: YOU HAVE A NEW PANTRY!

We purged our pantry and filled it with great new healing foods, supplements, cookware, and more. Now it's time to cleanse. The food cleansing protocol ahead is the wellness tool that has had the most *profound* transformation on my life and on the lives of my clients as well.

PART III:
EVERYDAY RADIANCE

Chapter 9

THE 21-DAY TRANSFORMATIONAL FOOD CLEANSE

The doctor of the future will give no medicine,
but will instruct his patient in the care of the human frame,
in diet and in the cause and prevention of disease.

- THOMAS EDISON

Rewind to 2007. Nearly every client I've guided has started their transformational journey with a food cleanse. I learned about the power of cleansing and detoxing in 2007 when I worked at Golden Cabinet, a very prominent integrative medical health center in Los Angeles, which was frequented by some of Hollywood's biggest, brightest, and most talented celebrities, writers, producers, CEOs, musicians, and business owners.

I came to realize that each and every person who walked through the door was a human being. It didn't matter whether they were a top celebrity, stay-at-home-mom or dad, or busy business owner. They were all there for a health check and to take a stand for their highest well-being. The experience dramatically changed my life.

I must admit that when I first began working as the medical center's in-house nutritionist and heard the word *cleanse* before it was as popular as it is today, it kind of freaked me out. I didn't know what it truly meant to cleanse or how I was going to feel.

Since the 21-day cleanse program was a cornerstone of the medical center, and since I was going to coach clients through it, I needed firsthand experience. Learning more about the healing benefits of detoxing and eliminating certain inflammatory foods from a science-based perspective gave me the confidence I needed, and I dove in.

HERE'S WHAT I EXPERIENCED

After a few days of changing my diet and adding customized supplements and a medical-grade shake designed to help my body rid itself of toxins and heavy metals, I felt better than I had in years. It's almost as if a veil lifted from my brain. I could see clearer. My energy soared and my body began to release unwanted weight and bloat. I also noticed my moods were better and my outlook on life was beginning to become more positive as well.

Honestly, the 21-day plan was pretty much miraculous. Once I completed it, I was committed to my health in a new way and I began coaching clients through the process. My goal from that point forward was to help each and every person I counseled achieve their own positive experience. Truthfully, I witnessed miracles.

As I worked with patients and clients over the next months and years, it became very clear that some loved the ease of the plan, while others struggled with rigid restrictions. For some, it was too steep a gradient or too much change at once. They needed smaller steps to begin. In an effort to make the plan easier for clients to stick with it and still get the tremendous results available to them, I modified it and created my own proprietary 21-day cleanse food plan, which I've been using in my practice ever since.

In this chapter, I outline the 21-day plan I have successfully used in my practice. This plan, tweaked and upgraded with the times as needed, has resulted in tremendous life-changing success for the people I coach and counsel. This success includes weight loss, less bloat, banished migraines, getting off medications, better sleep, a better functioning and more efficient metabolism, happier moods, greater energy, better digestion, more confidence, and better relationships too!

THE MAIN PILLARS OF
THE FOOD CLEANSE PLAN ARE:

1. Improve gastrointestinal health
2. Decrease body fat
3. Incorporate phytonutrients to improve estrogen detoxification
4. Improve estrogen metabolism
5. Reduce inflammation and balance blood sugar levels

Special Note: Before you begin the transformational food cleanse, I suggest you consider getting a blood test, as outlined in Chapter 4. A full blood panel helps you know your starting point. It's not necessary, though it is a helpful tool.

RENEW. REPAIR. REVITALIZE.

One of the aims of a food cleanse is to create a fresh start.

We want to up our game and feel healthier. While our goal is to create an abundantly healthy life, we want to focus on eliminating the foods that cause inflammation in the body. And we want to look at how much sugar we are eating. If the quantities are high, even the good forms of sugar found in fruits and starchy veggies can have a negative impact.

Experience a lighter, brighter, more confident you.

RADIANT TIP

WHAT'S YOUR WHY?

Taking back the power of your health starts with figuring out your WHY. Why do you want to feel better? Why do you want to lose the weight? You've got the high school reunion, your son's big event, your daughter's graduation. But what about the big picture? Do you want to live to see your kids get married? Or know your grandchildren? Take that European vacation you've always dreamed about? Or, finally unleash your passion and create that thriving business you know is inside of you waiting to be born? If so, these things take energy. They take good health. Knowing your WHY will give you endless insights into more WHATs and HOWs. Connecting to your WHY will give you inspiration, motivation, and a reason to stay on course when you want to quit. So get clear on your WHY. And while you're at it, write it down.

PHASE 1: SUPPORT THE BODY'S OWN NATURAL DETOXIFICATION PATHWAYS

Because of its simplicity, low cost, and superior therapeutic results, detoxification through food and lifestyle choices is the most exciting tool in natural medicine. You will notice changes in your health almost immediately!

Our bodies naturally detoxify and balance themselves. It is only when our detoxification mechanisms become overloaded with dietary and environmental stressors that the process becomes less efficient and symptoms may surface.

Toxins can be internal and/or external in origin. Improper digestion and imbalances of the digestive tract result in metabolic by-products from certain bacterial strains, which create internal toxins. These internal toxins (aka endotoxins) negatively impact overall health both by their toxic nature and by compromising detoxification pathways.

Symptoms that may be relieved by following a detoxification program include:

- Digestive disorders
- Constipation
- Irritability
- Bad breath
- Headaches
- Brain fog
- Joint pain
- Fatigue
- Itchy skin
- Chemical sensitivities
- Skin rashes/allergies

What a carefully planned detoxification eating program offers you:

- Anti-aging effects
- Reduction of allergic symptoms
- Increased energy
- Greater motivation and creativity
- Weight loss
- Clearer skin and eyes
- Mental detoxification

FOR THE NEXT 21 DAYS:

You'll eat meat, seafood, poultry, and eggs; lots of vegetables and fruit; natural, healthy fats; fresh herbs and spices. This program is designed to have no slips, cheats, or special occasions—though if you do, all you need to do is get back on track at your next meal.

The no cheat thing isn't me playing tough nutritionist; it's grounded in the science of an elimination diet, during which you have to completely eliminate suspected triggers to evaluate them. (If you never eliminate them, how will you know if your life could be better without them?)

The food cleanse is also about keeping your promise/commitment to yourself. You committed to 21 days of becoming more aware of your health, habits, and relationship to food. I want you to honor your commitment.

THE BEYOND RADIANT
FOOD CLEANSE PLAN RULES

WANT THE PLAN TO CHANGE YOUR LIFE?

FOLLOW THE GUIDELINES 100%

1. **Be mindful of all types of sugar you consume.** Try your best to avoid

consuming any added sugar during the next 21 days. Read labels because companies sneak sugar into products, A LOT (as I mentioned in Chapter 5). If you absolutely must have a tad of sweetness, opt for manuka or raw honey, coconut sugar, monk fruit, or stevia.

2. **Do not consume alcohol in any form.** Again, if you find that you *must* have some alcohol, opt for vodka with fresh lime or biodynamic or organic red wine. Avoiding alcohol will give your body (and your liver and gut) a rest and allow you to see what life is like without it!

3. **Limit legumes.** If you desire to lose weight, consider limiting legumes.

4. **Limit grains.** Reducing grains can support better weight loss for some.

5. **Avoid additives.** Do not consume carrageenan, MSG, or added sulfites. **Read labels!**

6. **Avoid stepping on the scale.** Your cleanse is so much more than a weight loss plan. You are getting back in touch with your body's natural, internal signals and cues. Plus, you are reconnecting with your emotional and physical well-being.

WHAT YOU NEED TO REMEMBER
WHEN ON THE FOOD CLEANSE:

1. **You're here because you're ready for change.**

2. **This is a 21-day plan.** It's not hard. You can do it!

3. **Avoid cheating.** Watch what happens to your self-confidence levels.

4. **What you eat is always a choice.** You get to choose, and you never have to eat something you don't want to eat. That goes for dinner parties, restaurant outings, or special events. (If you know the food at the event will not be on your list, eat before you go.) Oh yeah, and you don't have to explain yourself or make any excuses either to friends or family. This is *your* body and *your* life. It's always a choice.

5. **You have the tools for advance planning.** I'm giving you the tools for meal-planning, grocery shopping, cooking, and dining out at healthy establishments. But you also have to take responsibility for your own program and progress.

6. **Keep in mind that habits take time to break.** The long-term rewards are worth it.

7. **Have fun, and enjoy the journey.** YOU can do this!

RADIANT TIP

DETOX-FRIENDLY FOODS

Include cruciferous vegetables, sea vegetables, herbs, spices, green tea, and sulfur-containing foods like onions and garlic. All of these foods help your liver detoxify.

RADIANT TIP

GUT-FRIENDLY FOODS

Include probiotic foods and dietary fibers in the form of lignans and insoluble fibers, such as flaxseeds, leafy greens, psyllium husks, and bran. Aside from helping with satiety and balancing blood sugar levels, these foods bind to estrogen in the digestive tract so it can be excreted properly from the body. (Refer back to Gut 101 page in Chapter 3.)

FOOD CLEANSE SUPPLEMENTS

The following supplements may assist with sugar cravings, weight loss, and better blood sugar balance. They are not necessary, though they can be helpful for some.

1. **Probiotic:** Use a professional-grade or high-quality probiotic and avoid fillers.
2. **Berberine:** This helps support blood sugar and sugar cravings.
3. **Digestive enzyme:** These are good for aiding digestion.

WHAT EXACTLY IS AN ELIMINATION DIET?

Originally created by the Institute of Functional Medicine, an elimination diet is a personalized lifestyle diet and a simple way to establish your own formula for greater health. Think of the elimination diet as the key that has the potential to unlock a treasure trove of data on how food makes you feel. In my nutrition coaching practice and in my own life, the elimination diet is my first line of approach when helping clients look and feel their best. It provides a new baseline for health. Testing for food sensitivities can be expensive and not always 100 percent accurate. The elimination diet allows you to see how the food you are eating (or not eating) affects you.

The elimination diet is designed as a detox food plan and especially supports liver and gut health. While we are going to eliminate top food allergens, we are also going to put things back in that are nourishing. We track symptoms over 21 days. This is a three-week commitment to yourself. (Of course, you can always begin with one or two weeks to start, though three weeks will give you more feedback.) The plan is meant to be a system, although you can tweak and tailor the plan, if you must. Just begin!

REMEMBER THESE THREE KEY PRINCIPLES

1. **Variety:** Eat a variety of foods from the what's in list.
2. **Rotate your foods:** Avoid eating the same foods every day.
3. **Rotate colors:** Colors give you different health benefits.

JENNIFER'S JOURNEY

From Headaches to Happiness

Jennifer, in her forties, had spent thirty years of her life with horrible migraine headaches. She'd been to every top doctor in the LA area and beyond. She'd also been taking quite a few medications, including trial medications, to support her headaches. Nothing worked long term.

In 2011, Jennifer came to see me. I asked her if anyone had spoken to her about the food she was eating, especially gluten. She shared that no one had ever talked to her about food. At the time, gluten was being lightly discussed, but the concept that some people may be gluten-intolerant wasn't yet mainstream. I put Jennifer on my 21-day transformational food cleanse with an elimination diet that took her off of gluten, dairy, and refined sugars.

Within a few weeks, Jennifer's migraines were gone! Nine years later, she still lives her gluten-free lifestyle and feels great.

I've worked with many clients where the wrong food for their bodies was the root of their ill health. Food is powerful. It truly has the potential to heal us or harm us.

CHANGE YOUR FOOD, CHANGE YOUR LIFE.

PRIMARY GUIDELINES

Although we've touched upon some of these guidelines in Chapter 5, I will share them with you again to remind you of the top inflammatory foods to avoid while on the food cleanse. By eliminating these foods for a short period of time, we give our body a break and we see how these foods make us feel when we add them back in.

1. **DAIRY:** Eliminate (or reduce) all dairy products, including milk, cream, cheese, cottage cheese, yogurt, butter, ice cream, and frozen yogurt. Avoid products like soy cheese, which are made with casein (a milk protein).

2. **MEATS AND FISH:** Eliminate (or reduce) fatty meats like beef (except grass-fed), pork, and veal. Acceptable choices are chicken, turkey, lamb, and cold-water fish such as salmon, mackerel, seafood, and halibut (if you are not allergic to or intolerant of these foods). Choose free-range meats whenever possible and wild fish over farm-raised.

3. **GLUTEN:** Eliminate any foods that contain wheat, spelt, rye, barley, or malt. Acceptable choices for most individuals are products made from rice, millet, buckwheat, nut flours, coconut flour, tapioca, and arrowroot.

4. **YEAST:** Avoid foods containing yeast or foods that promote yeast overgrowth (processed foods, refined sugars, cheese, commercially prepared

condiments, peanuts, and any fermented foods such as soy sauce, white vinegar, and alcoholic beverages).

5. **ALCOHOL AND CAFFEINE:** Avoid (or reduce*) alcohol-containing products, including beer, wine, liquor. Also limit* beverages containing caffeine, including coffee.

   *Note: If you want to keep coffee in your day, limit your intake to 1–2 cups in the morning. Organic is best.

6. **WATER:** Stay hydrated. Drink pure, clean, fresh water. Herbal tea and soup counts too.

RELAX. BREATHE. GO FOR WALKS.

Enjoy the change of season. Celebrate the beauty of a cold, wintry day, gentle spring afternoons, and a hot summer morning. This is a time for you to care for your unique self.

BEYOND RADIANT: 21-DAY EATING PLAN

WHAT'S IN. WHAT'S OUT.

ANIMAL PROTEIN

IN: Fish, seafood, wild game, lean lamb, chicken, turkey, grass-fed beef, eggs (opt for organic)

OUT: Pork, veal, sausages, cold cuts, canned meats, hot dogs

VEGETABLE PROTEIN

IN: Split peas, lentils, legumes tempeh, tofu (organic)

OUT: Soybean products, processed varieties (soy yogurt, processed isolated soy)

DAIRY SUBSTITUTES

IN: Nut milks such as almond, hemp, and coconut milk, unsweetened, and plant-based yogurt, unsweetened

OUT: Dairy, milk, cheese, cottage cheese, cream, yogurt, butter, ice cream, non-dairy creamers

VEGETABLES

IN: Preferably fresh, raw, steamed, sautéed, juiced, roasted

OUT: Corn, creamed vegetables

FRUITS

IN: Whole low-sugar fruits—opt for seasonal, fresh, or frozen berries, apples, pears, peaches, nectarines, cherries, lemons, limes; and eat smaller portions of these fruits: grapes (a handful), pineapple (½ cup), mango (½), banana (½), melon (1 cup)

OUT: Orange juice, canned fruit with added sugar

DRINKS

IN: Filtered water, green tea, herbal teas, yerba mate, seltzer or mineral water

OUT: Soft drinks (diet and regular), Crystal Light, drinks with added chemicals and sugar

OILS

IN: Cold-pressed olive, flaxseed, avocado, sesame, almond, pumpkin, walnut, and coconut oils, butter from grass-fed cows, ghee

OUT: Margarine, shortening, salad dressings with added chemicals and sugar, mayonnaise, spreads, all refined and processed oils

SWEETENERS

IN: Avoid, but if you must, have small amounts of coconut sugar, raw honey, monk fruit, stevia

OUT: Refined white/brown sugars, high fructose corn syrup, barley malt, agave

CONDIMENTS

IN: All spices: sea salt, pepper, basil, carob, cinnamon, cumin, dill, garlic, ginger, mustard, oregano, parsley, rosemary, turmeric, thyme, vinegar (apple cider, rice, or balsamic), coconut aminos, tamari sauce (wheat-free)

OUT: Chocolate (processed), ketchup, relish, chutney, soy sauce, barbecue sauce, teriyaki, any condiment with added chemicals or sugar

NUTS AND SEEDS

IN: Walnuts, sesame, pumpkin, sunflower, hazelnuts, pecans, almonds, hemp seeds, brazil nuts, macadamia nuts; the best choices are raw or sprouted; minimize consumption of cashews, as they are higher in sugar.

OUT: Peanuts, peanut butter (inflammatory and higher in mold)

NON-GLUTEN GRAINS AND STARCH

IN: Brown rice, millet, quinoa, gluten-free oats, amaranth, buckwheat

OUT: Wheat, corn, barley, spelt, kamut, rye, couscous, farro

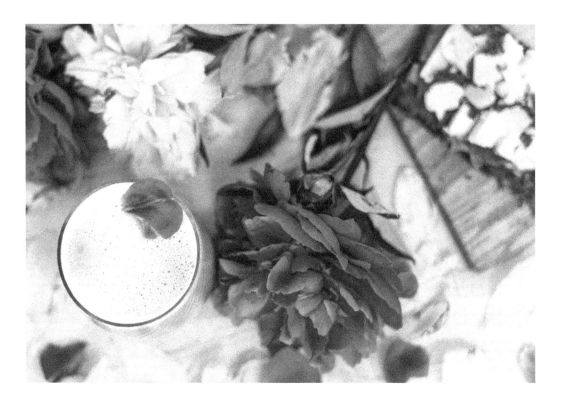

BEYOND RADIANT: SHAKES

These shakes and smoothies are loaded with simple ingredients to boost your beauty, balance your hormones, better your breast health, increase your energy, and sharpen your focus. Shakes are easy to make and incredibly delicious. Blend ingredients in a blender and enjoy.

THE BEYOND RADIANT BASIC SHAKE

- 1–2 scoops protein powder, plant-based (I love Epic and Sun Warrior brands)
- 1 tablespoon fiber (ground flax or chia seeds)
- 1 teaspoon healthy fat (medium chain triglyceride (MCT) coconut oil, plain extra-virgin coconut oil, or ¼ avocado)
- 1 cup almond milk, unsweetened (or other plant-based milk)

SIMPLE STRAWBERRY SHAKE

- 1–2 scoops protein powder
- 1 tablespoon fiber (ground flax or chia seeds)
- 1 cup almond milk, unsweetened
- ½ cup berries, fresh or frozen
- Dash of cinnamon

SOUTHERN STYLE SMOOTHIE

- 1–2 scoops protein powder
- 1 tablespoon fiber (ground flax or chia seeds)
- 1 cup almond milk, unsweetened
- ½ cup peaches, fresh or frozen
- 2 teaspoons freshly grated ginger
- Dash of cinnamon

VERY CHERRY PLEASURE

- 1–2 scoops protein powder
- 1 tablespoon fiber (ground flax or chia seeds)
- 1 cup almond milk, unsweetened
- ½ cup cherries, pitted, fresh or frozen
- 2 teaspoons nutmeg, freshly grated

CHOCOLATE BEAUTY KETO SHAKE

- 1–2 scoops, protein powder
- 1 tablespoon fiber (ground flax or chia seeds)
- 1 cup almond milk, unsweetened
- ¼ to ½ small avocado
- 1 tablespoon raw cacao
- Dash of cinnamon
- Few ice cubes for creaminess
- Optional: Dash of monk fruit for sweetness

RADIANTLY RASPBERRY

- 1–2 scoops protein powder
- 1 tablespoon fiber (ground flax or chia)
- 1 cup almond milk, unsweetened
- 1/2 cup raspberries, fresh or frozen
- Dash of cinnamon

OPTIONAL ADD-INS FOR ANY SHAKE:

- 1 teaspoon almond butter, unsweetened (for protein, healthy fat, and magnesium)
- 2 Brazil nuts, raw (for selenium, which supports thyroid health)
- 1–2 teaspoons hemp seeds (for extra protein)
- 1 handful raw spinach or kale (great for cleansing the body and blood)
- 1 tablespoon raw cacao powder (provides magnesium)
- 1 scoop collagen powder (great for beauty and joints)
- 1 teaspoon acai, powder or frozen (unsweetened)

HEALTHY FAT OPTIONS

These keep you fuller longer.

- 1 teaspoon coconut oil or MCT oil
- 1 teaspoon Brain Octane by Bulletproof
- 1 teaspoon to 1 tablespoon flax oil
- ¼ avocado
- 1 tablespoon coconut meat (whole)

METABOLISM BOOST

- 1 teaspoon matcha green tea powder

ADAPTOGENS:

- 1 teaspoon ashwagandha (stress reduction, calming)
- Pearl (beauty-boosting skin food!)
- 1 teaspoon reishi mushroom (immunity)
- 1 teaspoon rhodiola (brain and focus booster)
- 1 teaspoon cordyceps (energy)
- 1 teaspoon maca (energy, hormone balancing)
- 1 teaspoon amla powder (immunity, beauty)

A TOUCH OF SWEETNESS

- Coconut water, fresh
- 1 Medjool date

- 1 teaspoon of lucama powder or monk fruit

BEYOND RADIANT: SNACK SUGGESTIONS

ALL SNACKS BELOW ARE BASED ON THE FAT, FIBER, PROTEIN PHILOSOPHY.

These feature a variety of ways to incorporate avocados, nuts, nut butters, beans, hummus, berries, fruits, veggies and gluten-free crackers.

1. Salsa served with cut-up veggies (carrots, celery, jicama, pea pods) and ¼ avocado on the side, or toss avocado into the salsa. This is a quick and easy fun snack. Choose a salsa brand you like, or make your own. Salsa should be free of additives and preservatives.

2. ¼–½ an avocado mashed with sea salt, served with veggies (carrots, celery, jicama, cauliflower, etc.) and 5–8 flax crackers. (I love Mary's Gone Crackers.)

3. Avocado veggie hand rolls: Place ¼ to ½ mashed avocado, julienned carrots, cucumbers, cabbage, or any veggies you like on nori sheets. Top with sea salt, roll up into a cone, and enjoy! Two cones are a nice afternoon snack.

4. One whole small apple, sliced and served with 1 tablespoon almond butter. Sprinkle the apples and almond butter with cinnamon and a pinch of sea salt for a sweet and salty treat.

5. Raw veggie sticks (celery, carrots, jicama) dipped in 1 tablespoon raw almond butter or guacamole (Try Brenda's Famous Guacamole in the recipe section in Chapter 10.)

6. Two celery ribs with 1 tablespoon of almond butter.

7. ½ cup sliced mixed berries with 1 tablespoon almond butter.

8. 6–8 small rice crackers or 1 large rice cracker with 1 tablespoon almond butter.
   Optional: Drizzle cracker with raw honey and top with blueberries or cinnamon.

9. 5–7 gluten-free crackers with veggies and 1 tablespoon almond butter.
10. ¼–⅓ cup hummus (try Marlyn's Healthy Hummus in the recipe section in Chapter 10) with gluten-free or flaxseed crackers or veggies.
11. Small piece of fruit with 15–20 raw almonds, 7–8 walnuts, or 3 Brazil nuts.
12. Half-cup split pea, lentil, or black bean soup.

BEYOND RADIANT: BEAUTY FOODS

BONUS POINTS FOR EATING THESE HIGH-FIBER, HIGH-ANTIOXIDANT, HORMONE-BALANCING BEAUTY FOODS!

- Apples
- Arugula
- Beets and their greens
- Berries
- Broccoli
- Brussels sprouts
- Cacao (raw)
- Cauliflower
- Flaxseeds, ground
- Goji berries
- Green tea (try matcha!)
- Maca
- Persimmons
- Pomegranate
- Rooibos tea
- Sprouts (try broccoli, pea, or sunflower sprouts)
- Tulsi tea (holy basil)
- Yams

Note: The cruciferous family of vegetables, including broccoli, Brussels sprouts, and cauliflower, are especially good for supporting detoxification and clearing out unhealthy estrogens from the body. Try incorporating one or more servings a day or at minimum three to five times per week.

RADIANT TIP

FOOD AND LIFESTYLE DURING 21-DAY DETOX

- No fried foods!
- Stay hydrated. Enjoy succulent foods, soups, water, herbal teas.
- Make an oil change! Use olive oil in salad dressings.
- A shake is great for breakfast. Or try oatmeal or a veggie omelette.
- Add more greens to your day (salads, green juice, sautéed, or powders).
- Eliminate gluten, dairy, and refined sugars.
- Eat 1–2 servings of fresh, low-sugar, organic fruit per day.
- Add in healthy snacks (see snack suggestions).
- Eat small amounts of protein throughout the day.
- Become a food detective. **READ LABELS!**
- Intermittent Fasting: Try a 12–14 hour fast each night or a few times a week.
- Increase your sleep. Aim for 6–8 hours per night.
- Try a magnesium supplement or 1 teaspoon of almond butter for better sleep.
- Check labels for sugar, chemicals, and food additives.
- Take time to rest and relax.
- BREATHE. Be mindful of your breath throughout the day, so you can ground yourself in the moment.
- Move your body each day. Walk, hike, ride a bicycle, whatever you enjoy.
- Eat mindfully! Slow down and take time to chew your food.
- Take a few deep breaths before you eat. Aim for twenty-minute meals.

21 WAYS TO CREATE
A HEALTHIER LIFESTYLE

CHOOSE ONE (OR MORE!)
OF THE TIPS BELOW TO FOCUS ON EACH WEEK.

LIFESTYLE RITUALS: PICK ONE OR MORE
TO TRY DURING AND AFTER THE CLEANSE.

1. Meditate. Even if you begin with 3–5 minutes per day, make room for morning me time.
2. Get a massage.
3. Declutter. (A drawer, a room, or your closet!)
4. Dry brush your skin with a dry body brush, found at most health food stores and online. (Opt for a medium-firm plant-based brush.) Dry brushing is a great way to exfoliate old skin cells and create a more youthful glow. Always brush skin toward the heart.
5. Detox your kitchen.
6. Upgrade your cosmetics, beauty, hair, and facial products. Begin to switch your products to cleaner, chemical-free varieties.
7. Go for a walk or hike. (Turn your phone off!)
8. Try yoga. (Try restorative yoga for relaxation.)
9. Breathe using 7+7+7. (Inhale, hold, release, for 7 seconds each.)
10. Sleep. Go to bed half hour to an hour earlier than usual. Or, take a 15–20 minute power nap!
11. Steam/Sauna. In the shower, alternate between hot and cold water. This wakes up the body and is therapeutic for many. It's good for the lymphatic system and circulation.

    TIP: Take your normal shower. At the end of your shower consider turning up the hot water to where it's tolerable. Let it rinse all over you. Then turn the cold water down to where it's tolerable. Repeat this three to seven times.
12. Use salt scrubs, or add ½ cup Epsom salts to your bath.
    (Very good for extra detox support.)
13. Shop at a farmer's market.

14. Use nontoxic cleaning products at home.

15. Experiment with essential oils for relaxation.

16. Create an afternoon or evening tea ritual before bed.

17. Try grounding. Walk barefoot on the earth, or at the beach. This is energizing.

18. Create a morning ritual with lemon water or green tea and slow 7+7+7 breathing.

19. Consider a Sunday night dinner ritual with family and/or friends to enjoy healthy food and conversation. Potluck works too.

20. Take 3 long, slow deep breaths before each meal to create presence.

21. Have a green juice. Try celery or another green veggie drink. It's great for cleansing the blood.

Chapter 10

THE RECIPES

You don't have to cook fancy or complicated masterpieces—just good food with fresh ingredients.

\- JULIA CHILD

This section is filled with an array of wellness-inspired recipes to help calibrate metabolism, balance blood sugar, boost sex drive, heighten focus, increase energy, harmonize hormones, improve sleep, inspire beauty, and support weight loss. All recipes can be used during and after the 21-Day Cleanse.

Whether you want to step up your cooking game for friends or family, learn a few new recipes for your girls' night in, or simply get back into the kitchen to take care of YOU in a healthy new way, think of cooking as a therapeutic, playful, fun, sensual art.

In 2009, I was feeling uninspired to cook. My friend Romy invited me to join her in a cooking class in LA at a cool new vibey place called Hipcooks. Hipcooks's philosophy is all about bringing playfulness back to cooking and to have us fall in love with the magic of prepping, peeling, baking, and creating. Hipcooks encourages you to leave the rest behind, especially the perfection. Measuring implements are banned and you're welcome to taste while you cook, so you can assess what a dish might need—perhaps a pinch of cumin, a dash of cayenne pepper. In the months that followed, I took a variety of cooking classes, including their Thai, Indian, Italian, Mediterranean, and gluten-free and dairy-free desserts classes. It was super fun and inspirational! You could say that my inner chef came alive. Honestly, it reminded me of being with my Susie Homemaker toy oven as a kid (which I LOVED!) and transformed my relationship with cooking, entertaining, and creating in the kitchen.

So go ahead, follow the recipes as suggested, or make up your own as you go. Cooking is one thing in your life you can control. You can add, tweak, or modify where needed. Whatever feels good. Have fun as you play and create, and treat your body well.

TINY TIPS AND HELPFUL GUIDELINES

Organic: I recommend using organic ingredients whenever possible.

Gluten: If you have celiac or are gluten sensitive, check brand packages to see if they are made in a facility with other products containing gluten.

Vanilla: When the recipe calls for vanilla, opt for sugar-free varieties. Look for organic and/or real vanilla bean.

Cinnamon: Ceylon cinnamon is an excellent variety that tastes great and helps to balance blood sugar. Consider using it when a recipe calls for cinnamon.

DRINKS AND ELIXIRS

I love visiting healing spas and healthy food markets.
I also love a great women's health retreat!
With a little prep, planning, and imagination,
we can bring the beauty of a serene spa and
health-inspired market into our own homes
through wellness-inspired lattes,
tonics, and elixirs.

GOLDEN MILK LATTE

SERVES ONE.

Calming, healing, and delicious, this caffeine-free, immune-boosting, anti-inflammatory turmeric latte is the perfect morning drink or evening delight.

INGREDIENTS

- 1 cup almond milk, unsweetened, or other plant-based milk
- 1½ teaspoons organic ground turmeric
- ½ teaspoon black pepper

PREP

1. Set your burner to medium. In a small saucepan, combine the almond milk, turmeric, and black pepper. Whisk together for a few minutes until hot.
2. Pour into your favorite mug, let cool slightly, and serve.

Alternately, steam the milk with a steamer. Transfer to a blender and add the turmeric and black pepper. Blend on high speed until frothy.

CHOCOLATE REISHI LATTE

SERVES 1

A chocolatey, hormone-balancing drink that soothes the mind and calms the nervous system, while also providing energy and metabolism-boosting essentials, this warming elixir was inspired by Erewhon foods. It's the drink I introduce my clients to when I take them on a shopping tour. Reishi is known as the queen of mushrooms. It's an adaptogenic, medicinal mushroom that helps to enhance the immune system, reduce stress, and support deeper, more restful sleep. Reishi has a woodsy, earthy taste, and when paired with cacao, cinnamon, and almond milk, it makes for a beautiful, healing, tasty tonic.

INGREDIENTS

- 1 cup of tulsi holy basil tea, warm
- 1/4 cup almond milk, unsweetened
- 1 teaspoon coconut oil
- 1–2 teaspoons cacao powder, raw
- 1/2 teaspoon reishi powder
- Cinnamon to taste
- Optional: raw honey, coconut sugar, or stevia to taste

PREP

1. Make the tea and let it steep for about 5 minutes.
2. Warm or steam the almond milk.
3. Place the tea, almond milk, coconut oil, cacao powder, reishi powder, cinnamon, and optional sweetener in a blender, and blend until frothy.
4. Pour into your favorite mug. Enjoy.

ROOIBOS RADIANCE TEA

SERVES 1

This caffeine-free tea elixir is loaded with antioxidants and earthy vanilla notes from the rooibos leaf. The tea supports digestion, inner calm, and overall well-being. Drink anytime, day or night. I especially love it in the evening before bed. Add a bit of manuka honey for a true healing adventure.

INGREDIENTS

- Rooibos tea (tea bag or loose leaf tea)
- 1 teaspoon manuka (15+ or 24+) honey
- 1 cup hot water

PREP

1. Place the tea bag in hot water in a teapot, or in a French press if using loose tea.
2. Add Manuka honey.
3. Let steep for a few minutes.
4. Pour the tea into your favorite mug.
5. Sip, savor, and enjoy!

MACA HOT CHOCOLATE ELIXIR

SERVES 1

This sensual, delicious, hormone-balancing hot chocolate is infused with the ancient healing powers of maca and cinnamon. Plus, it's got just the right amount of heat from the cayenne pepper. With its natural libido-boosting and metabolism-enhancing qualities, it's sure to set your body, blood, and brain on fire—in a good way! Double up the recipe and share with your special someone.

INGREDIENTS

- 1 cup almond milk, or other plant-based milk
- 1–2 tablespoons raw cacao powder
- 1 teaspoon maca powder
- ¼ teaspoon cinnamon
- 1 teaspoon MCT oil
- Pinch Himalayan pink sea salt
- Pinch cayenne pepper (optional)
- 1 teaspoon coconut sugar or monk fruit to sweeten (optional)

PREP

1. Heat plant-based milk on the stovetop until hot (avoid boiling).
2. Place the milk in a blender. Add the cacao powder, maca powder, cinnamon, MCT oil, Himalayan sea salt, optional cayenne powder, and coconut sugar
3. Blend until well combined. You can also use a hand frother.
4. Sip, savor, and enjoy!

MARLYN'S MATCHA LATTE

SERVES 1

A favorite of my clients, this gorgeous go-to morning (or afternoon) drink is perfect when you want a boost of caffeine without the coffee. Matcha is known for its cancer-kicking, estrogen-detoxifying, and blood-enhancing ingredients, like ECGC, chlorophyll, and L-theanine. It's a great boost for the metabolism, mood, and brain.

INGREDIENTS

- 1 cup almond, coconut, or other plant-based milk
- 1 teaspoon matcha green tea powder
- 1 teaspoon MCT oil
- ¼ teaspoon cinnamon

PREP

1. Place the plant-based milk, matcha green tea powder, MCT oil, and cinnamon in a pot.
2. Heat until warm.
3. Pour mixture into the blender and pulse on high for 30 seconds until frothy. You can also use a hand frother.
4. Serve in your favorite mug and enjoy!

RADIANT TIP

Add ¼ teaspoon of pearl powder to your matcha tea for radiant skin that glows.

GINGER IMMUNITY TONIC

SERVES 1

This soothing, healing, and calming-to-the-senses tonic is loaded with vitamin C from the fresh lemon and anti-inflammatory properties form the fresh ginger. Manuka honey is also known for its digestive, antibiotic, and antiviral effects. Consider drinking in the morning or anytime you need an immunity boost.

INGREDIENTS

- 1 cup of hot water
- ¼ lemon, fresh
- 3 slices of fresh ginger, ¼ inch each
- 1 teaspoon of Manuka honey (optional)

PREP

1. Squeeze the fresh lemon into the hot water.
2. Add the ginger slices and optional Manuka honey to the hot water.
3. Let sit for 2–3 minutes.
4. Sip slowly and enjoy.

BREAKFAST

MARLYN'S RASPBERRY MUFFINS

MAKES 12 MUFFINS

Simple, delicious, and naturally sweet, these high-powdered, antioxidant-filled muffins are loaded with gut-healing fiber and plenty of beauty-boosting ingredients like berries, flaxseeds, and cinnamon. They're sure to hit the spot when you crave a healthy, nourishing treat. Consider making an extra batch and freeze the leftovers for breakfast or an anytime snack. Great topped with your favorite nut butter or served warm with a drizzle of raw honey.

INGREDIENTS

- 2 ½ cups almond flour
- ½ teaspoon baking soda
- 2 teaspoons ground cinnamon
- 3 tablespoons ground flaxseeds
- ½ cup coconut sugar, monk fruit, or raw honey
- ½ cup water

- 3 eggs
- ¼ teaspoon pure vanilla extract or pure vanilla bean powder
- 2 tablespoons coconut oil
- 1 ½ cups raspberries (or other berries)

PREP

1. Preheat the oven to 350°F.
2. Line muffin tins with paper wrappers.
3. In a small bowl, combine almond flour, baking soda, cinnamon, flaxseeds, and monk fruit or coconut sugar. (If using honey, add in step 4.)
4. In a separate bowl, whisk together water, eggs, vanilla, and honey (if using). Pour the wet ingredients into the dry ingredients and mix well.
5. Add the coconut oil.
6. Gently fold berries into the batter.
7. Use an ice cream scoop to fill each baking cup ¾ full with the batter.
8. Bake for 20–25 minutes or until golden brown.

Extra Protein: You can add 2 scoops of protein powder (or collagen) to the batter if you want even more muscle-building protein. A great pre-workout meal.

BEYOND RADIANT NUT AND SEED BREAD

MAKES 1 LOAF

This simple nut and seed bread, loaded with fiber (including gut-healing psyllium husk) and other healthy ingredients, is an all-time favorite and inspired by the nut and seed bread at Breadblok bakery on Montana Avenue in Santa Monica. I first tasted their delicious gluten-free, dairy-free bread at the Studio City Farmers Market. From my first bite, I was hooked. Make the recipe as is, or play with the ingredients and design them to please your own taste buds.

INGREDIENTS

- ½ cup raw almonds, whole, with skins
- 1 ½ cups rolled oats
- 1 cup sunflower seeds
- ½ cup ground flaxseeds
- ¼–½ cup raisins

- 2 tablespoons coconut oil
- 1 teaspoon sea salt
- 3 tablespoons psyllium husk
- 1 tablespoon 100% maple syrup
- 1½ cups water

PREP

1. Place all the ingredients in a bowl and knead them until combined.
2. Let the mixture sit for 2 hours in the refrigerator.
3. Preheat the oven to 350°F.
4. Place the mixture into a 9 x 5 bread pan, pressing the ingredients down so the top is smooth and even.
5. Bake for 20 minutes.
6. Carefully remove the bread from the pan.
   Turn the bread over and fit it back into the pan.
7. Bake the bread for another 30 minutes.
8. Place the pan on a plate and let cool.
9. Once the bread has completely cooled, you can slice it and use as you would use regular bread. Nut bread stays fresh on your countertop for about three days, in your fridge for a month, and up to a year in the freezer.

ROSEMARY PUMPKIN MUFFINS

MAKES 8 MUFFINS

If you love pumpkin like I do, these power-packed, fiber-filled muffins are sure to satisfy your pumpkin palate. Loaded with immune-boosting vitamins and minerals like vitamin A and magnesium, plus healthy feel-good fats, they're the perfect breakfast companion or afternoon energy boost.

INGREDIENTS

- 1 cup almond flour
- 2 tablespoons coconut flour
- 1 ½ teaspoons baking powder
- ¼ cup raw pumpkin seeds, divided
- 3 large eggs

- 1 cup pumpkin puree
- 2 teaspoons fresh rosemary leaves, chopped, or ¾ teaspoon dried rosemary
- Coconut oil for greasing muffin tins

PREP

1. Preheat the oven to 350°F.
2. Lightly grease 8 cups in a muffin tin with coconut oil. Set aside.
3. In a medium bowl, whisk together the almond flour, coconut flour, plus 3 tablespoons pumpkin seeds.
4. In a separate bowl, whisk together the eggs, pumpkin purée, and rosemary.
5. Stir the wet ingredients into the dry ingredients until fully incorporated.
6. Divide the batter among prepared muffin cups and sprinkle with the remaining pumpkin seeds.
7. Bake until a wooden toothpick inserted into the center of a muffin comes out clean, about 30 minutes. Let the muffins cool in the pan for a few minutes before transferring them to a plate or rack to cool completely.

PUMPKIN BREAKFAST COOKIES

MAKES 20 COOKIES

Plenty of healthy fats, fiber, and plant-based protein make these pumpkin cookies the perfect on-the-go breakfast or healthy snack. They're brimming with beautiful, warming spices like cinnamon and nutmeg and skin-boosting vitamin A for a gorgeous, illuminating glow.

INGREDIENTS

- 1 ½ cups almond flour
- 1 teaspoon baking soda
- 2–3 teaspoons pumpkin pie spice
- 1 teaspoon cinnamon
- ¼ teaspoon nutmeg
- ⅓ cup unsweetened coconut flakes
- 1 tablespoon chia seeds, soaked in ¼ cup of water for 10 minutes
- ½ cup pureed pumpkin
- ½ cup almond butter

- 1 tablespoon vanilla extract
- ¼ cup maple syrup (if on cleanse, substitute monk fruit powder)
- 1 tablespoon freshly grated ginger, or ½ teaspoon powdered ginger
- ½ cup walnuts, broken into small pieces
- ½ cup dried goji berries or dried tart cherries, unsweetened

PREP

1. Preheat the oven to 375° F.
2. In a large bowl fitted for an electric mixer, combine the almond flour, baking soda, pumpkin pie spice, cinnamon, nutmeg, and unsweetened coconut flakes. (If on the cleanse, add monk fruit powder.) If using dried ginger, add now. Make a small well in the middle of the dry ingredients and add the chia seeds with any liquid, pureed pumpkin, almond butter, vanilla, maple syrup, and fresh ginger, if using. Set the mixer on medium-low and thoroughly combine.
3. Add the walnuts and dried berries. Gently incorporate using a large spoon.
4. Line a baking sheet with parchment paper and spoon the cookie dough onto the sheet, 2 inches apart. Bake for 12–15 minutes, and let cool.
5. Store in the refrigerator or freeze for a longer shelf life.

BETTER FOR YOU BANANA BREAD

SERVES 8

Banana bread! Need I say more? Loaded with wholesome ingredients, this fragrant, sweet, dense loaf gives you nourishment and pleasure without the energy-depleting, refined sugar crash. Great for a mid-morning snack, afternoon bite, or a quick-and-easy travel treat. Bake an extra loaf and share it with your BFF, colleague, or that special someone in your life.

INGREDIENTS

- 2 ripe bananas, mashed
- ⅓ cup coconut sugar (if on cleanse, omit sugar, or add monk fruit)
- ¾ cup almond milk, unsweetened
- ¼ cup coconut oil
- 1 egg

- 2 teaspoons vanilla extract
- ¾ cup coconut flour
- ¾ cup almond flour
- 2 teaspoons baking powder
- ½ teaspoon sea salt
- 1 teaspoon ground cinnamon

Optional add-ins:

- ¾ cup unsweetened dark chocolate chunks
- ¾ cup fresh blueberries

- ½ cup of whole walnuts for top of bread

PREP

1. Preheat the oven to 350 °F.
2. Lightly grease a 9 by 5 loaf pan with coconut oil.
3. In a large bowl, thoroughly combine the mashed bananas, coconut sugar, almond milk, coconut oil, egg, and vanilla.
4. In a separate bowl, mix together the coconut flour, almond flour, baking powder, salt, and cinnamon.
5. Fold the dry ingredients into the wet ingredients. Mix until the wet ingredients are completely incorporated.
6. Gently fold in the chocolate chunks or blueberries, if desired.
7. Pour the batter into the loaf pan. Scatter the walnuts over the top, if desired.

8. Bake for about 55–60 minutes, or until a toothpick inserted in the center comes out clean.

9. Let the bread cool for 10 minutes.

10. Invert the bread onto a heatproof plate or wire rack and continue to cool. Bread is delicious when still warm.

SUPERFOOD WILD BERRY MUESLI

SERVES 1

This beauty-boosting, gut-healing, grain-free muesli makes a great power breakfast or mid-morning snack. It travels well too. Simply pack muesli in small containers or baggies. Pack fresh fruit in a separate container, or add dried fruit to the muesli mix. Bring a carton of your favorite plant-based milk. To make your life easier, you can also omit the milk and use water. Or add your favorite adaptogens for a mind-body boost. (See one of my favorite combinations below.)

INGREDIENTS

- ½ cup uncooked rolled oats
- 1–2 tablespoons raw nuts (walnuts, sliced almonds, or cashews)
- 1 tablespoon unsweetened coconut flakes (optional)
- 1 tablespoon ground flaxseeds
- ¼ teaspoon cinnamon
- 1–2 dried figs (no sulfites), cut up in small pieces
- ½ cup fresh blueberries, blackberries, strawberries, or raspberries; or ¼ cup dried blueberries, blackberries, strawberries, or raspberries
- ½ cup coconut, almond, soy, or other plant-based milk, unsweetened

PREP

1. In a cereal bowl, combine the oats, nuts, coconut flakes, flaxseeds, figs, and fresh blueberries, blackberries, strawberries, or raspberries.
2. If making the muesli for travel, substitute dried fruit for fresh.
3. Top with the coconut or almond milk.
4. Stir to combine, and enjoy.

NOTE: For overnight oats, make the muesli, add the milk (or water), cover, and store in the fridge until morning.

ONE OF MY FAVORITE MUESLI COMBINATIONS

½ cup oatmeal, 1 teaspoon maca, 1 teaspoon raw cacao, ¼ teaspoon turmeric, ¼ cinnamon, ¼ teaspoon raw honey, 1 ½ cups boiling water. Soak for five minutes. Top with flaky sea salt.

WINTER WARMING GRAIN-FREE PORRIDGE

SERVES 2

This warming bowl of nourishment is packed with plenty of healthy fiber, warming spices like cinnamon, cardamom, and vanilla, and gorgeous amounts of plant-based protein too. Makes a great power breakfast or hormone-balancing midmorning snack.

INGREDIENTS

- 1 tablespoon pumpkin seeds
- 2 tablespoons shredded unsweetened coconut
- 2 teaspoons chia seeds
- ½ teaspoon cinnamon
- ¼ teaspoon cardamom
- 1 teaspoon vanilla bean powder
- ¼ teaspoon pink Himalayan sea salt
- Hot water to cover

- 1 teaspoon raw honey, 1 teaspoon maple syrup, or 1 teaspoon monk fruit *(optional)*
- ½ pear or apple, chopped
- 1 tablespoon goji berries or dried figs, chopped into small pieces
- Coconut milk, almond milk, or other plant-based milk, unsweetened

PREP

1. Using a hand blender or food processor, process the pumpkin seeds, coconut, chia, cinnamon, cardamom, vanilla, and sea salt until finely ground.
2. Place mixture in a serving bowl, and add ground flaxseeds.
3. Add hot water to cover.
4. Add sweetener of choice, and mix well.
5. Top with pear or apple, dried fruit, and a drizzle of plant-based milk.
6. Let sit for 2–3 minutes to absorb liquid.

RADIANT TIP

Double down! Make a double batch of dried ground seeds and store in a glass jar in the refrigerator to eat later in the week.

SOUPS

BEYOND RADIANT CARROT GINGER SOUP

SERVES 4–6

Simple, pure, and incredibly delicious, this anti-inflammatory, skin-enhancing soup is loaded with vitamin A from polyphenols and immune-boosting extra-virgin olive oil, ginger, and rosemary. Great for immunity and lung health. Think of this soup as health in a bowl.

INGREDIENTS

- 2 tablespoons extra virgin olive oil
- 1 medium onion, chopped
- 2 cloves garlic, crushed
- 1 teaspoon ground rosemary
- 1 teaspoon ground ginger, or 1 tablespoon fresh ginger, finely chopped
- 3 cups carrots, peeled and chopped (6 large or 8 medium)
- ¼ cup fresh parsley, chopped
- Sea salt and pepper to taste
- 4 cups organic vegetable stock or water
- 1 bunch fresh cilantro (or other herbs), chopped

PREP

1. Heat the oil in a large pot until it shimmers.
2. Add the onions, garlic, and rosemary, and sauté until the vegetables are soft.
3. Add the carrots, parsley, ginger, salt, and pepper and sauté for 2–3 minutes
4. Pour in the vegetable stock and bring to a boil.
5. Cover and simmer for 30 minutes, or until the carrots are very soft.
6. Remove from heat and let the soup cool for five minutes
7. Using an immersion blender or high-speed blender, puree the soup until smooth. If the soup's consistency is too thick, add more vegetable stock.
8. Adjust seasonings to taste, heat through, ladle into bowls, and sprinkle with cilantro or other fresh herbs before serving.

COSMIC CUCUMBER AND AVOCADO SOUP

SERVES 2

Simple, refreshing, and creamy, this incredibly satisfying soup tastes like spring in a bowl. Loaded with gorgeous amounts of vitamins C and E and healthy fats to enhance beauty, glow, and cell rejuvenation, this soup makes the perfect lunch when you want something quick, easy, and decadent without the fuss. A great addition for a girlfriend get-together lunch.

INGREDIENTS

- Zest of 1 lime
- Juice of 2 limes
- 1 teaspoon sea salt
- 2 medium cucumbers, peeled and seeded, roughly chopped
- 1 avocado, peeled, pitted, and roughly chopped
- Parsley, cilantro, rosemary, or thyme (or a mix of your favorite herbs), chopped

PREP

1. Place lime zest, lime juice, sea salt, cucumbers, and avocado in a deep bowl or high-speed blender.
2. In the bowl, blend with an immersion blender until the soup is creamy.
3. In the blender, set speed to medium-high and pulse until the soup is creamy.
4. Divide soup between two bowls, and scatter herbs over each.

SIMPLY ROASTED ASPARAGUS SOUP

SERVES 2

Layered with feel-good fat, fiber, and a touch of fresh garlic, this immune-boosting, age-defying soup is sure to hit the spot and keep you healthy, happy, and hormonally balanced all day long. Great for a relaxing evening meal, or paired with a nice salad and a gluten-free pumpkin muffin. (See pumpkin muffin recipe later in this chapter.)

INGREDIENTS

- 1 bunch asparagus, cut into bite-sized pieces
- 3 tablespoons extra virgin olive oil, divided
- 2 cloves garlic, roughly chopped
- 1 leek, cleaned and roughly chopped
- 4 cups vegetable broth or water
- Sea salt and freshly ground pepper to taste
- 1 tablespoon chopped chives

PREP

1. Preheat the oven to 350°F.
2. In a medium bowl, add the asparagus and coat with one tablespoon of the olive oil. Place the asparagus on a foil-lined sheet and roast for 10 minutes until just tender.
3. Meanwhile, in a pot over medium heat, add the remaining olive oil, garlic, and leek. Coat the garlic and the leek thoroughly with the oil. Reduce the heat to medium-low and sauté the garlic and leeks, stirring them frequently until the garlic is fragrant and the leeks become soft and translucent.
4. Add the asparagus and the broth.
5. Bring the soup to a boil, then reduce heat to simmer.
6. Simmer soup for 10 minutes to marry the flavors.
7. Turn off the heat. With an immersion blender, blend the soup so that it's smooth and creamy. Or, cool the soup for five minutes and pour into a high-speed blender. Pulse at medium-high until creamy.
8. Taste and add sea salt and freshly ground pepper.
9. Top with chives, serve, and enjoy.

RADIANT TIP

Add a dash of cayenne pepper for an extra bit of heat and metabolism boost.

LONGEVITY ZUCCHINI SOUP

SERVES 4–6

With an array of healing herbs, spices, and gorgeous gut-healthy veggies like garlic, onion, and zucchini, this delicious soup will leave you energized, beautified, and feeling happy and uplifted. Great for lunch, or pair it with your favorite salad, gluten-free muffin, or one of the main courses ahead.

INGREDIENTS

- 1–2 tablespoons extra virgin olive oil
- 2 cloves garlic, crushed
- 1 medium onion, chopped
- 4 zucchini, diced
- 4 cups vegetable stock or water
- Sea salt and freshly ground black pepper to taste
- 1 tablespoon fresh herbs (basil, oregano, cilantro)

PREP

1. Heat the olive oil in a soup pot.
2. Add the chopped onion and crushed garlic.
3. Sauté the vegetables until they are soft.
4. Add the zucchini and sauté for another 2–3 minutes.
5. Add the stock, salt, and pepper. Bring to a boil.
6. Reduce heat, cover, and simmer until the zucchini are tender.
7. Add fresh herbs.
8. When the soup is cool, puree it with an immersion blender, or in a conventional blender until smooth.
9. Reheat before serving.

BUTTERNUT SQUASH AND PEAR SOUP

SERVES 6

Savory, satisfying, and delicious, this beauty-enhancing soup will hit the spot any time you crave a bowl of healthy, sweet goodness. Infused with warming spices like cardamom and cinnamon plus immunity-building, skin-hydrating ingredients like vitamins A, C, and E, it will serve as a lovely addition to your autumn, spring, or winter wellness plan.

INGREDIENTS

- 2 pounds butternut squash, peeled, seeded, and cut into ¾" dice, about 4 cups
- 6 ripe but firm pears, peeled, cored, and cut into ¾" dice, about 4 cups
- 3 tablespoons olive oil, divided
- 3 tablespoons fresh-squeezed orange juice, divided
- ¼ teaspoon sea salt, or to taste

- ½ cup water, divided
- ⅓ cup chopped shallots
- 2 tablespoons Madras curry powder
- ¼ teaspoon ground cardamom
- 6 cups vegetable broth or water
- 1 stick cinnamon, 2 inches
- Fresh herbs (cilantro, rosemary, or thyme) for garnish

PREP

1. Preheat the oven to 400°F.
2. On a large baking sheet, toss the squash and pears with 2 tablespoons of the oil and 2 tablespoons orange juice until well coated. Season with the salt.
3. Drizzle with two tablespoons of water.
4. Roast the squash and pears until tender, approximately 30–40 minutes. Add more water, if necessary, to prevent burning.
5. When the squash and pears are tender, remove 1 cup. Set aside and save for garnishing the soup.
6. In a large soup pot over medium-low heat, add the remaining tablespoon of olive oil. Add the shallots and sauté, stirring often so they become soft, but not brown.
7. Add the remaining tablespoon of orange juice, the curry powder, and the cardamom. Cook for 2 minutes.

8. Add the remaining squash and pears.

9. With an immersion blender, or in batches with a conventional blender, puree mixture until smooth. If using a conventional blender, pour mixture back into pot. Add the broth and the piece of cinnamon stick. Bring to a simmer. Reduce the heat to low and simmer for 25–30 minutes, stirring occasionally. Season with the salt and pepper, if desired. Discard the cinnamon stick.

10. Top each bowl of soup with a sprinkling of the reserved squash and pears.

11. Garnish the soup with the fresh herbs and a drizzle of olive oil.

BEAUTIFUL BROCCOLI SOUP

SERVES 6–8

Broccoli is a girl's best friend. The magical cruciferous vegetable is loaded with natural estrogen-detoxifying properties and cancer-kicking ingredients. When you add potent plant polyphenols from fresh garlic and thyme, this wonderful soup is a true bowl of goodness that will leave you feeling energized and optimized. Broccoli has a constituent called sulforaphane, which is immune-boosting and antiviral. This soup is great for dinner, lunch, or an afternoon snack.

INGREDIENTS

- 1 tablespoon extra virgin olive oil
- 1 medium onion, chopped
- 2 cloves garlic, crushed
- 2 pounds broccoli, rinsed and chopped
- 1 teaspoon ground thyme
- Sea salt and freshly ground pepper to taste
- 6–8 cups organic vegetable stock (depending on how thick you want your soup)
- Fresh chopped parsley or other herbs of choice (chives and dill are nice)

PREP

1. In a large pot over medium heat, add the oil, onion, and garlic. Sauté until the onion is soft and translucent.
2. Add the broccoli, thyme, sea salt, pepper, and stock. Bring to a boil.
3. Cover, reduce heat, and simmer until the broccoli is tender, about 40 minutes.
4. Check and adjust seasoning.
5. Puree the soup with an immersion blender or cool for five minutes and whirr in a high speed blender. Garnish with fresh herbs.

SALADS

ASIAN CARROT-AVOCADO SALAD WITH GINGER DRESSING

4–6 SERVINGS.

A delicious, refreshing salad infused with the beautiful flavors of ginger, cilantro, and sesame seeds. This crunchy, wellness-inspired salad will tantalize your taste buds and fill your body with plenty of fiber, fresh vegetables, and healthy fats. Makes a great lunch or light evening meal.

INGREDIENTS

For the salad:

- 4 cups carrots, grated
- ½ cup cilantro, chopped
- ½ cup parsley, chopped
- ½ cup raw sesame seeds (set aside 2 tablespoons for garnish)
- 1 medium avocado, chopped

For the dressing:

- 2 tablespoons extra virgin olive oil or flaxseed oil
- 3 tablespoons fresh lime juice
- 1 ½ tablespoons tamari
- 1 tablespoon fresh ginger, minced, or ½ teaspoon dried ginger
- ½ teaspoon ground coriander
- 1 teaspoon coconut nectar or honey (optional)

PREP

1. In a large bowl, toss the carrots with the cilantro, parsley, and sesame seeds. Set aside.
2. In a food processor, blend the oil, lime juice, tamari, ginger, coriander, and coconut nectar (or honey).
3. Pour the dressing over salad, and toss well.
4. Gently fold in the avocado, and sprinkle reserved sesame seeds over the salad before serving.

CHINESE CHOPPED SALAD

SERVES 4–6

Gorgeous, colorful vegetables loaded with minerals, antioxidants, and plant-based polyphenols enliven this beautiful salad. It's also infused with anti-inflammatory ginger, sesame, and olive oil for an age-defying delight. Think of this chopped salad as an illuminating beauty treatment in a bowl.

INGREDIENTS

For the salad:

- 4 cups Chinese cabbage, shredded
- 6 cups romaine lettuce, shredded
- ¼ cup scallions, white and green parts
- 1 cup snow peas
- 2 cups mung bean sprouts
- ¾ cup almonds (raw or roasted), sliced or chopped½ cup goldenberries (also called gooseberries)

For the dressing:

- 2 ½ tablespoons tamari or coconut aminos
- 1 ½ tablespoons apple cider vinegar
- 2 tablespoons fresh squeezed orange juice
- ¼ cup extra virgin olive oil
- 1 tablespoon plus 1 teaspoon fresh ginger, grated
- 1 whole red jalapeño pepper, minced (with or without seeds; seeds will add heat)¼ cup sesame seeds, toasted

PREP

1. In a large bowl, toss the Chinese cabbage, romaine lettuce, scallions, snow peas, mung bean sprouts, almonds, and goldenberries until well combined. Set aside.
2. To make the dressing, place the tamari, apple cider vinegar, orange juice, and olive oil in a glass measuring cup or a nonreactive bowl. Whisk together until combined. Add the ginger, jalapeño, and sesame seeds. Whisk thoroughly.
3. Pour the dressing over the salad, toss gently, and serve.

SPRING MIXED GREENS
WITH GOJI BERRY DRESSING

SERVES 2

An array of tastes and textures makes this salad fun, satisfying, and delicious. I also love the natural sweetness and anti-aging benefits of the dressing.

Goji berries are naturally infused with resveratrol, which is known to support immunity and good health. In traditional Chinese medicine, goji berries are highly regarded as a medicinal herb that supports liver, eye, and lung health.

INGREDIENTS

For the salad:

- 2 cups mixed spring greens (arugula, spinach, lettuce mix)
- ¼ cup shredded beets
- ¼ cup shredded carrots
- 1 fennel bulb, thinly sliced
- Chopped fresh spring herbs (fennel leaves, mint, cilantro, oregano)
- Fresh sprouts (broccoli, radish, sunflower)

For the dressing:

- 2 tablespoons fresh orange juice
- 3 teaspoons apple cider vinegar
- ½ cup extra virgin olive oil
- ¼ cup water
- 1 clove garlic, finely chopped, or 1⁄2 teaspoon garlic powder
- ½ teaspoon sea salt
- ½ cup goji berries, soaked in water for 1–2 hours, or until soft
- ¼ cup cilantro

PREP

1. Place the spring greens, beets, carrots, fennel bulb, spring herbs, and sprouts in a serving bowl. Toss until combined. Set aside
2. To make the dressing, in a blender, place the orange juice, apple cider

vinegar, olive oil, water, garlic, salt, goji berries, and cilantro. Blend until well combined.

3. Fold the dressing into the salad. Transfer to a platter, and serve.

Flavorful goji berry dressing can be used with any other salad of choice. Its natural sweetness from orange juice and rich antioxidant ingredients from goji berries and cilantro makes this dressing the perfect accompaniment to the tender greens and crunchy vegetables.

RADIANT TIP

For an extra protein boost, top the salad with sliced grilled organic chicken breast or wild-caught shrimp or tuna. You can also make an extra batch of dressing. Store it in a glass jar for use later in the week.

CURRIED TUNA SALAD
IN BUTTER LETTUCE LEAVES

SERVES ONE.

INGREDIENTS

- 1 six-ounce can tuna (preferably wild-caught)
- ½ stalk celery, chopped into small pieces
- 1–2 teaspoons Dijon mustard
- ¼ cup parsley, finely chopped
- 1–2 teaspoons curry powder
- Sea salt and pepper
- 3 large lettuce leaves, washed and dried (butter lettuce works especially well)
- 6 cucumber slices

PREP

1. Drain the tuna and place in a bowl.
2. Use a fork to flake the tuna.
3. Add the celery, mustard (to your taste), parsley, and curry powder (to taste).
4. Mix the ingredients well, and season with a little sea salt and freshly ground pepper.
5. Scoop an equal amount of the tuna mixture into each lettuce leaf.
6. Top each with two cucumber slices.
7. Roll up and eat.

MEDITERRANEAN QUINOA SALAD

SERVES 4

This longevity-promoting, nutrient-dense salad brims with the fresh flavors of the Mediterranean. Follow the recipe as is, or mix and match the nuts, vegetables, and dried fruits listed below to create your own tasty version. Serve as a main course or a side dish. For a heartier version, add your favorite high-quality proteins, like organic free-range chicken, grass-fed beef, or wild-caught salmon, tuna, or shrimp. Great for a luncheon, intimate dinner party, or healthy evening family get together.

INGREDIENTS

For the salad:

- 2 teaspoons olive oil
- 1 cup quinoa
- 2 cups organic vegetable stock or water
- 1 teaspoon sea salt
- 1 cup cherry tomatoes or mini heirloom tomatoes, cut in half
- 2–3 small Persian cucumbers, sliced thin
- 1 cup pine nuts, toasted
- 2 tablespoons sesame seeds, toasted
- 5 basil leaves, rolled lengthwise into cigar shapes and thinly sliced

For the dressing:

- 2 cloves garlic, minced
- Juice of 2 lemons
- ½ teaspoon fresh lemon zest
- ¼ teaspoon sea salt
- ¼ teaspoon ground cumin
- 2–3 tablespoons fresh orange juice
- 1 cup extra virgin olive oil

PREP

1. In a medium saucepan, heat 2 teaspoons of olive oil until the oil shimmers. Add the quinoa. Sauté for 2–3 minutes, or until the quinoa smells nutty.

2. Add the water or the vegetable broth and the sea salt. Stir to combine.

3. Turn heat up to high and bring the mixture to a boil. Once the water boils, turn the heat to low and cover the saucepan with a lid. Cook for 20 minutes.

4. Remove the pan from the heat and let the quinoa stand for 5 minutes.

5. While the quinoa cooks, prepare the dressing. In a mixing bowl or measuring cup, add the garlic, lemon juice, lemon zest, sea salt, cumin, and orange juice. Whisk to combine.

6. Slowly add the olive oil, whisking until the dressing is mixed thoroughly. Set aside.

7. Lift the lid from the pan holding the quinoa (be mindful of steam rising up), and fluff the quinoa with a fork. Transfer the quinoa to a glass bowl.

8. Once the quinoa has completely cooled, add the tomatoes, cucumbers, pine nuts, sesame seeds, and basil. Toss to combine.

9. Drizzle the citrus dressing over the quinoa and gently incorporate.

10. Transfer the quinoa salad to a platter. Serve at room temperature.

RADIANT TIP

Get creative. Consider adding additional ingredients according to your tastes and desires. Here are some ideas:

- Dried fruits: figs, raisins, dried cherries, currents
- Toasted nuts or seeds: almonds, walnuts, pecans, pumpkin seeds
- Roasted vegetables; broccoli, cauliflower, butternut squash, red or yellow peppers
- Fresh herbs: rosemary, thyme, cilantro, parsley, mint
- Spices: cinnamon, cardamom, turmeric, nutmeg, cayenne pepper

(Recipe courtesy of Culinary Bliss LA)

BRENDA'S FAMOUS GUACAMOLE

Each time I venture from Los Angeles to New York City to visit my soul sister Brenda, she has delicious healthy food waiting for me. Her food satisfies my hunger, soothes my spirit, and tantalizes my senses. (Think warm blanket, big hug, and a mother's love all wrapped in one.) One of Brenda's all-time favorite specialties is her homemade guacamole. I asked Brenda to share her recipe.

This guacamole can be chunky or smooth depending on how you like it. To me, what makes the guacamole so delicious is the quality and ripeness of the ingredients. Enjoy! Love, Brenda

INGREDIENTS

- 3 ripe avocados, lightly soft to the touch but not mushy, pitted, peeled and mashed
- Finely chopped red onion, to taste (approximately 2 teaspoons1/2 ripe plum tomato, diced 1 teaspoon sea salt, or to taste
- Pinch of fresh cilantro, chopped (optional)

PREP

1. In a medium bowl, mash together the avocados and the sea salt.
2. Mix in the onion, tomatoes, and cilantro (optional).
3. Refrigerate for 1 hour for best flavor, or serve immediately.

MARLYN'S HEALTHY HUMMUS

This quick, easy, and delicious hummus is packed with monounsaturated fats, protein, vitamins, minerals, and antioxidants. Great for an afternoon pick-me-up or salad accompaniment.

INGREDIENTS

- 1 15 ½ ounce can organic chickpeas with liquid
- ½ cup tahini paste
- 1 clove garlic, crushed
- ¼ cup lemon juice
- ¾ teaspoon pink Himalayan sea salt
- Drizzle of olive oil
- ¼ cup chopped parsley, for garnish

PREP

1. In a food processor, add the chickpeas with all their liquid, the tahini paste, garlic, lemon juice, and salt.
2. Process the ingredients on medium-high until smooth and light, about 2 to 3 minutes.
3. Taste and adjust for seasoning.
4. Spoon the hummus evenly into a shallow serving bowl. Drizzle with the olive oil and scatter the top with parsley.
5. Serve with cut-up veggies or gluten-free crackers like Mary's Gone Crackers.

MORE SALAD IDEAS

It's of great benefit to eat a fresh green salad with your lunch or evening meal. Think of greens as blood cleansers, liver cleansers, beauty enhancers, and gut-healers. To make your salad, combine the following and dress with one of the dressings in the salad section:

Choose different kinds of lettuces:

- Arugula*
- Belgian endive
- Butter lettuce
- Cabbage (red, green, Napa, Savoy)
- Curly endive
- Dandelion*
- Mesclun
- Mustard greens
- Radicchio
- Red leaf lettuce
- Romaine
- Spinach
- Watercress*

Top your salad with at least 4 different fresh veggies:

- Avocado*
- Beets,* steamed or grated
- Broccoli, raw
- Carrots, raw or gently steamed
- Celery*
- Cucumber
- Fennel bulb,* chopped or sliced
- Herbs, chives, parsley,* oregano, mint, cilantro,* dill, etc.
- Radishes*
- Seeds (raw sunflower, pumpkin, or sesame seeds)
- Snap peas
- Spring onions
- Sprouts*

The items marked with an asterisk are known for their detoxifying properties.

RADIANT TIP

COOKING AND PREP WORK TIPS

1. I know from personal experience that it's a lot easier to make good snack and meal decisions if you have good choices readily available. Take the time to chop, cut, or buy precut celery, carrots, bell peppers, cucumbers, jicama, etc., so you have a snack ready to go when you have a snack attack and it would be too easy to reach for cookies or chips. Store your veggies in a glass container in the fridge for longer freshness. You can also blanch green beans or asparagus to keep in your fridge for snacking. Dip your veggies in a little tahini, hummus, or guacamole for a delicious fat, fiber, and plant-protein treat.

2. Make a big pot of greens that are ready to go any time. Set a pot of water to boil. Clean your greens, pull of the stems, and tear into smaller pieces. Once the water boils, drop in the pieces. Turn off the heat, and cover. Let sit for 2 minutes. Drain and store.

    Blanched greens will keep for about a week in your fridge. You can also precut some of the heartier vegetables like fennel, shiitake mushrooms, and most of the greens to make evening cooking quicker. Just store them in glass containers in the fridge.

3. If you like to drink green juices but don't have the time to make them every day, you can make a double batch and pour half into a glass jar. Green juice usually keeps for about three days.

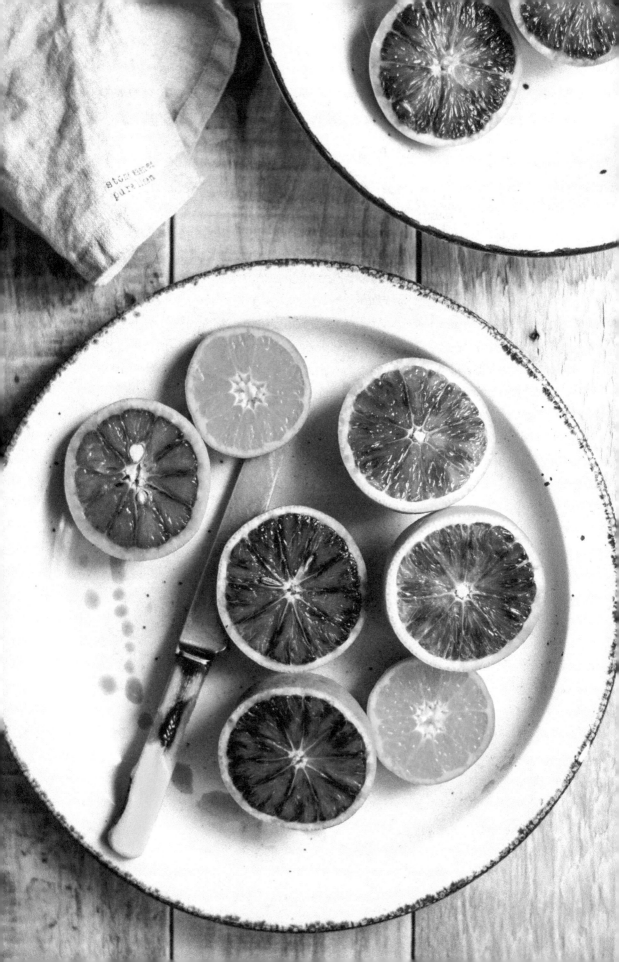

ADDITIONAL DRESSINGS

BASIC SALAD DRESSING

A great dressing to have available anytime you want a healthy zing to your salad.

INGREDIENTS

- 4–6 cloves garlic, chopped
- 1 tablespoon Dijon mustard
  or 1 teaspoon dry mustard powder
- 1 large handful parsley, washed,
  dried, and roughly chopped
- ⅔ cup apple cider vinegar
- ⅓ cup extra virgin olive oil
- Sea salt and pepper to taste

PREP

1. Put all the ingredients in a glass jar with a lid.
2. Shake vigorously until ingredients are thoroughly mixed.
3. Taste and adjust seasonings to your personal preference.
4. Store in the fridge for up to 2 weeks.
5. You may need to shake the dressing each time you use it.

BLOOD ORANGE DRESSING

MAKES ABOUT 1 CUP

INGREDIENTS

- 4–6 cloves garlic, chopped
- 1 tablespoon Dijon mustard or 1 teaspoon dry mustard
- ⅓ cup blood orange juice (about 1–2 oranges)
- 1 large handful parsley, washed, dried, and roughly chopped
- ⅓ cup apple cider vinegar
- ⅓ cup extra virgin olive oil
- Sea salt and pepper to taste

PREP

1. Put all the ingredients in a glass jar with a lid.
2. Shake vigorously until the ingredients are thoroughly mixed.
3. Taste and adjust seasonings to your personal preference.
4. Store in the fridge for up to 2 weeks.

FRESH LEMON VINAIGRETTE

MAKES ABOUT 1 CUP

INGREDIENTS

- 1 clove garlic, crushed (optional)
- ¼ cup freshly squeezed lemon juice
- ¾ cup extra virgin olive oil
- ¼ teaspoon sea salt
- Freshly ground black pepper to taste (optional)

PREP

1. Put all ingredients in a glass jar with a lid.
2. Shake vigorously until ingredients are thoroughly mixed.
3. Taste and adjust seasonings to your personal preference.
4. Store in the fridge for up to 2 weeks.
5. You may need to shake the dressing each time you use it.

MAINS

PAN ROASTED WILD SALMON WITH FRESH PESTO

SERVES 4

INGREDIENTS

- 3 cloves garlic
- 1-½ cups fresh basil leaves
- ½ cup Italian parsley
- Zest of half a lemon
- Sea salt and freshly ground black pepper
- ¼ cup olive oil, plus extra for rubbing onto fish
- 4 6-ounce salmon fillets, preferably wild-caught

PREP

1. Preheat the oven to 350°F.
2. Place garlic cloves in the bowl of a food processor or blender, and process until minced.
3. Add basil leaves, parsley, lemon zest, and a pinch of sea salt and pepper, and process again until all herbs are minced.
4. Slowly add the oil and process until pesto is smooth.
5. Heat a medium-sized skillet over medium-high heat.
6. While the pan is heating, brush the salmon fillets with the olive oil.
7. Sprinkle the filets with sea salt and pepper.
8. When the pan is hot, place the salmon into the pan, flesh side down.
9. Brush the top of each piece of salmon with some of the pesto sauce and cook for 3 minutes.
10. Carefully flip the fillets. Brush with more of the pesto sauce.
11. Transfer the salmon onto a baking sheet and put into the oven. Cook for an additional 3 to 4 minutes.
12. When the salmon is cooked through, remove from the oven, and transfer to a serving platter.

(Recipe courtesy of Culinary Bliss LA)

HEALTHY HEMP PESTO

You can substitute this flavorful pesto made with hemp nuts, rich in potassium and iron, for the pesto in the recipe above.

INGREDIENTS

- ½ cup fresh basil leaves, firmly packed
- ½ cup raw hemp nuts
- ⅓ cup flaxseed oil or extra virgin olive oil
- 1 teaspoon mashed garlic (about 2–3 cloves)
- ¼ teaspoon sea salt

PREP

Combine basil leaves, hemp nuts, oil, garlic, and salt in a food processor and blend until well incorporated

SIMPLE ROASTED
WILD SALMON

SERVES 2

INGREDIENTS

- 2 wild-caught salmon filets,
  4–6 ounces each
- Juice of ½ lemon
- 2 tablespoons coconut aminos
- Sea salt and freshly ground pepper

PREP

1. Set your oven's broiler to medium-high.
2. Place the salmon on a baking sheet.
3. Season the salmon with a little sea salt and pepper, then pour lemon juice and coconut aminos over the top of the fish and let sit for 10 minutes.
4. Place salmon on a rack set 2–3 inches under your broiler.
5. Keep an eye on the pan to make sure the fish doesn't burn.
6. Broil for 8–10 minutes. Salmon is ready when it flakes easily and has turned a light pink color.

(Recipe courtesy of Culinary Bliss LA)

BAKED SALMON WITH AVOCADO AND MANGO SALSA

SERVES 2

INGREDIENTS

For the salmon:

- 2 wild-caught salmon filets, 4–6 ounces each
- Juice of 2 lemons
- 4 teaspoons coconut oil
- Sea salt and pepper

For the salsa:

- 1 medium red onion, diced
- 1 avocado, cut into ¼–½ inch cubes
- ½ cup mango, cut into ¼–½ inch cubes
- 4 teaspoons cilantro, chopped fine
- 2 teaspoons green chili, seeded and minced
- 1 teaspoons garlic, crushed or finely chopped

PREP

1. Preheat the oven to 325°F.
2. Grease the bottom of a heavy baking pan or oven-safe skillet with the coconut oil.
3. Brush both sides of the salmon steak with the lemon juice and place the salmon in the baking dish or skillet.
4. Sprinkle the fish with the sea salt and pepper.
5. Bake the fish for 10–15 minutes or until its flesh is moist and flaky.
6. While the fish is cooking, prepare the salsa.
7. In a medium bowl, combine the onion, mango, avocado, cilantro, and chili.
8. In a small bowl, mix together the lime juice and the macerated garlic. Sprinkle the lime-garlic mixture over the salsa and toss.
9. Spoon the salsa over the baked fish, and serve.

CARIBBEAN ROASTED HALIBUT WITH PAPAYA SALSA

SERVES 2

INGREDIENTS

For the halibut:

- 2 tablespoons lemon or lime juice
- 2 teaspoons olive oil
- 1–2 tablespoons fresh cilantro or Italian parsley, rough chopped
- 2 halibut filets, 4 ounces each (or any other fresh fish you enjoy)

For the salsa:

- 2 cups diced ripe papaya
- 2 tablespoons minced red onion
- 1 avocado, diced
- 1–2 cloves garlic, chopped

PREP

1. Preheat the oven to 400°F.
2. In a medium bowl, whisk together the citrus juice, olive oil, and cilantro or parsley.
3. Line a sheet pan with heavy-duty foil or parchment paper and place the halibut fillets on the pan. Drizzle 1 tablespoon of the citrus dressing onto each piece of fish.
4. Add the papaya and red onion to the remaining dressing and toss gently to combine. Set aside.
5. Turn the preheated oven up to broil at medium-high.
6. Place the pan in the oven and broil fish for about 6 to 8 minutes, checking to make sure the fish doesn't burn.
7. If the fish starts to burn, turn off the broiler and set the oven to 350°F. Continue to cook the fish until it starts to flake and becomes opaque in the center.
8. Before serving the fish, gently add the avocado to the salsa. Carefully transfer the fish to plate or platter, and spoon the salsa over the fish.

CHICKEN WITH ASPARAGUS AND SUN-DRIED TOMATOES

SERVES 2, WITH LEFTOVERS FOR 1 LUNCH

Through the years, I've led many online and in-person wellness workshops and events. During my first online program in May 2012, I teamed up with Cardio Barre Fitness Studios to create the Body Bliss 21-Day Detox Challenge. This cutting-edge program was one of the first of its kind. We launched the program six times over the course of two years and had a total of 750 participants. While creating the Body Bliss Challenge, I asked my colleague Julia Sarver to design an array of healthy, simple-to-make recipes to accompany the plan. Many of her recipes are featured here. This one was a crowd favorite.

INGREDIENTS

- ⅔ pound boneless, skinless, free-range, organic chicken breasts, cut into small chunks
- ½ onion, chopped
- 4 garlic cloves, minced
- 1 bunch asparagus, tough ends snapped off and cut into 1-inch pieces
- 10 cremini mushrooms, trimmed, wiped clean, and cut into quarters
- 2 tablespoons sun-dried tomatoes in oil (sulfite-free), cut into small pieces
- Sea salt and freshly ground pepper

PREP

1. Heat a large skillet over medium-high heat.
2. Add the olive oil, chicken, and onion to the pan and cook until the chicken begins to brown.
3. Add the garlic and mushrooms and cook a few minutes more.
4. Add the asparagus and the sun-dried tomatoes and cook until the asparagus is bright green and still crisp.
5. Crack some freshly ground pepper over the top, and serve. Let each person add sea salt, if needed.

SESAME CHICKEN WITH BROCCOLI, GINGER, AND GARLIC

SERVES 2

INGREDIENTS

- 2 heads of broccoli cut into pieces, approximately 2 cups
- 4 tablespoons sesame oil
- 8 ounces boneless chicken, thinly sliced
- 4 tablespoons ginger, minced
- 2 cloves garlic, minced
- 4 tablespoons wheat-free tamari
- Sesame seeds for garnish

PREP

1. In a large pot, add 8 cups of water and a pinch of sea salt. Bring the water to a simmer.
2. Place the broccoli in the water and cook the broccoli until tender (test with a fork), roughly 2–3 minutes.
3. Remove the broccoli from the water and cool. Set aside.
4. Heating a wok or sauté pan over medium-high heat.
5. Add the sesame oil and the chicken pieces, stirring so that the chicken doesn't burn.
6. Add the ginger and garlic.
7. Add the blanched broccoli and tamari.
8. Cover and allow the chicken and broccoli to steam for 2–3 minutes.
9. Spoon the chicken and broccoli into a large bowl and top with sesame seeds before serving

PHIL'S CHICKEN PESTO

SERVES 2

My friend Phil, a master in the kitchen, shared this recipe with me. Phil's recipes are loaded with taste, flavor, and fresh ingredients from his Italian New York family roots.

INGREDIENTS

- 2 ½ cups basil leaves
- 2 cloves garlic, sliced
- 2 tablespoons lemon juice
- 1 teaspoon lemon zest
- 2 tablespoons olive oil
- 4 teaspoons coconut oil
- 2 chicken breasts, 4 ounces each
- Sea salt and pepper, if desired

PREP

1. Preheat the oven to 425°F.
2. In a food processor or blender, blend the basil, garlic, lemon juice, and lemon zest.
3. Slowly pour the olive oil into the blender and combine. Add the coconut oil and whirr until the ingredients are fully emulsified.
4. Place the chicken on a rimmed baking pan or shallow baking pan. Add salt and pepper, if desired.
5. Coat the chicken with the pesto mixture.
6. Bake chicken until cooked through, about 30 minutes

LEMONY CHICKEN SKEWERS

SERVES 4

INGREDIENTS

- Juice from 1 lemon
- 1 tablespoon olive oil
- 1 tablespoon fresh oregano, finely chopped
- 1 pound boneless, skinless, organic chicken breasts
- Sea salt and fresh ground pepper

PREP

1. Turn on the grill and set the heat to medium-high.
2. In a bowl, whisk together the lemon juice, olive oil, and oregano. Set aside.
3. Cut the chicken into 1-inch chunks and thread the pieces onto metal or wooden skewers. If using wooden skewers, be sure to soak the skewers in water for 10 minutes to avoid burning them.
4. Season the chicken with salt and pepper. Grill for 6–8 minutes, turning halfway through.
5. Chicken is done when the juices run clear.
6. Alternately, bake the chicken skewers in a 375°F oven for 10–12 minutes, turning once or twice, or sauté in a skillet on the stove.
7. When chicken is cooked, remove the meat from the skewers and toss it in the lemon juice mixture. Serve immediately.

BROWN LENTIL DAL

SERVES 2

Rich with traditional Indian spices and flavors and authentically cooked to perfection, this is a beautiful healing dish for body, mind, and spirit.

INGREDIENTS

- 1 tablespoon olive oil
- 2 cloves garlic, minced
- 1 medium yellow onion, chopped
- 1 cup small, brown lentils
- ½ cup cooked large red kidney beans, rinsed and cut in half

- 1 cup tomatoes, chopped
- Juice of ½ lemon
- 1 ½ teaspoons fresh ginger, minced
- Freshly ground pepper

PREP

1. Heat the olive oil in a medium-sized saucepan.
2. Sauté the garlic and the onion until soft.
3. Add the lentils, curry powder, and salt.
4. Add the water and bring the mixture to a boil. Lower to a simmer and cook for 30–40 minutes until the lentils are soft.
5. Add the kidney beans and tomatoes and cook for another 5–10 minutes.
6. Stir in the lemon juice. Add salt to taste.
7. Simmer the daal on the stovetop for another 5–10 minutes until all flavors are beautifully blended.
8. Serve with brown rice, basmati rice, or quinoa.

COCONUT VEGETABLE CURRY

SERVES 2–4

INGREDIENTS

- 1 yellow onion, chopped
- 1 clove garlic
- 1 tablespoon fresh ginger, chopped
- 1 green chili, seeded
- 1 tablespoon coconut oil
- ½ teaspoon turmeric
- ½ teaspoon coriander
- 1 teaspoon curry powder
- 1 each red, yellow, and orange pepper, chopped
- ½ head of cauliflower, chopped
- 1 carrot, chopped
- 1 zucchini, cut into cubes
- 1 cup coconut milk
- ½ teaspoon sea salt, or to taste

PREP

1. Process the onion, garlic, ginger, and chili in a food processor until smooth.
2. In a large skillet, add the coconut oil, the onion mixture, the turmeric, coriander, and curry powder.
3. Cook for 1 minute.
4. Add the peppers, cauliflower, carrot, zucchini, and coconut milk. Stir well.
5. Add sea salt to taste.
6. Cover and cook for 20 minutes until vegetables are tender.
7. Serve with brown rice, basmati rice, or quinoa.

SAUTÉED ZUCCHINI RIBBONS WITH GARLIC AND SHALLOTS

SERVES 2

INGREDIENTS

- 1 pound zucchini or fresh zucchini noodles
- 1 ½ tablespoons olive oil
- 1 teaspoon minced shallots

- 2 cloves garlic, minced
- 2 teaspoons lemon juice, fresh
- Sea salt and pepper

Option: Toasted pine nuts or hemp seeds for topping

PREP

1. With a noodle device, make the zucchini noodles. Or slice the zucchini lengthwise on a hand grater or a mandolin. (Note: You can also use sliced zucchini noodles from your favorite market.)
2. In a large nonstick skillet, heat the olive oil over medium heat.
3. Add the shallots and sauté until golden brown.
4. Add the garlic, and cook for another 30 seconds.
5. Turn the heat up to medium-high and add the zucchini noodles, sea salt, and pepper.
6. Cook, tossing and stirring the zucchini for 2 to 3 minutes until the zucchini softens.
7. Add a bit more sea salt and freshly ground pepper, as desired.
8. Top with toasted pine nuts or a sprinkle of hemp seeds.

(Recipe courtesy of Culinary Bliss LA)

SIDES

SIMPLE GARLIC BROCCOLI

SERVES 2

INGREDIENTS

- 1 large head broccoli and its stalk, tough outer layer removed, cut into even-sized chunks
- 2 tablespoons water
- 4 garlic cloves, thinly sliced
- Olive oil
- Sea salt and pepper to taste

PREP

1. Heat a skillet over medium-high heat.
2. Add the broccoli and water to the skillet. Bring to a boil and reduce to simmer.
3. Cover with lid, and allow the broccoli to steam for 3–4 minutes.
4. Add the garlic, toss with the broccoli, and continue to cook until the broccoli is bright green and still crisp.
5. Remove from heat and drizzle a little olive oil over the top.
6. Season with sea salt and pepper, and serve.
7. As an alternative, try drizzling the broccoli with olive oil and roasting it in the oven at 400°F for 10–15 minutes.

RADIANT TIP

The stem is often the tastiest part of broccoli, but it's important to first peel the stem or cut away the tough outer skin. Try peeling the stem of broccoli like a carrot and the stem may become your new favorite snack!

SESAME GREENS STIR-FRY

SERVES 2

INGREDIENTS

- 4 cups mixed greens (collards, arugula, spinach, or kale), tough stems removed
- 3 garlic cloves, thinly sliced
- 2 tablespoons hot water
- 1 teaspoon olive oil
- ½ teaspoon apple cider vinegar (optional)
- Toasted sesame seeds

PREP

1. Heat a skillet over medium-high heat and add the greens, garlic, and hot water.
2. Stir the greens so the hot water hits all the leaves, tossing for 3–5 minutes until the greens become bright green and cooked through.
3. Remove from heat and drizzle with the olive oil and vinegar.
4. Top with toasted sesame seeds.

ROASTED JAPANESE YAMS
WITH A HINT OF CINNAMON

SERVES 4

The sweet Japanese yam, also known as the mountain yam, marries well with the warming taste of cinnamon, a combination that helps keep insulin levels in check. A distant relative of the potato, Japanese yams provide protein, thiamin, vitamin C, and healthy starch. Enjoy with a variety of other vegetables for a beautiful plant-based meal or pair with a protein and green salad. When selecting Japanese yams, look for evenly sized, thinner yams.

INGREDIENTS

- 1 ½ pounds Japanese yams, about 4
- ¼ cup olive oil
- ¾ teaspoon Himalayan sea salt
- ¾ teaspoon cinnamon

PREP

1. Preheat the oven to 400°F.
2. Line a baking sheet with foil or baking paper.
3. Scrub and cut the yams into 1-inch coins. If you have larger yams, cut them in half lengthwise and cut each half into 1-inch moons.
4. Place the yams in a large bowl. Toss the yams with the olive oil until they are evenly coated.
5. Spoon the yams onto the baking sheet in a single layer. Sprinkle the yams with salt and cinnamon. Bake for 20 minutes. Remove the tray from the oven and turn over the potatoes. Continue baking for an additional 15 to 20 minutes, making sure the potatoes are nicely browned, but do not burn.
6. Remove the potatoes from the oven. Loosen from the pan and serve.

TREATS AND SNACKS

KRUNCHY KALE CHIPS WITH SEA SALT

SERVES 2

INGREDIENTS

- 1 bunch kale (curly green or purple)
- 2 tablespoons olive oil
- Juice of ½ lemon
- 1 teaspoon sea salt

PREP

1. Preheat the oven to 400°F.
2. Wash the kale thoroughly, and let dry.
3. Hold the bottom of the stem with one hand. With the other, use your thumb and forefinger to pull the kale up and away from the stem.
4. Gently tear the kale into smaller chip-size pieces.
5. Place the kale, olive oil, lemon juice, and salt into a bowl and massage all ingredients together with your hands.
6. Lay the massaged kale out on a baking sheet.
7. Place in the oven and set the timer for 15 minutes.
8. At 15 minutes, remove the kale from the oven, stir gently, place back in the oven, and bake for another 10–15 minutes until the kale is crispy and slightly golden brown.
9. Allow the kale chips to rest on the baking sheet and cool completely.
10. Store in an airtight glass container for 2–3 days.

ADDITIONAL TOPPINGS

Create a wave of playfulness. Up your kale chip flavors with a dash of cayenne pepper, hot paprika, curry powder, garlic powder, or everything blend from Trader Joe's.

AUTUMN-BAKED SWEET POTATO CHIPS

SERVES 4

When it comes to a satisfying snack, meal, or accompaniment, these baked sweet potato chips—sweet and crunchy with a touch of salt and bursting with lots of gut-healing fiber and skin-boosting vitamins A and C and B vitamins—will surely hit the spot.

INGREDIENTS

- 2 medium sweet potatoes (or yams), scrubbed, thinly sliced
- 1 tablespoon olive oil or melted extra virgin coconut oil
- ¼ teaspoon of sea salt

PREP

1. Preheat the oven to 350°F.
2. Place the sweet potatoes, olive oil, and salt into a bowl.
3. With your hands, evenly coat the potatoes with olive oil and salt.
4. Lay the sweet potatoes on a sheet pan lined with foil or parchment paper. Make sure the potatoes don't touch one another.
5. Bake the potatoes for about 12 minutes.
6. Remove the tray from the oven and flip each chip. Return the tray to the oven.
7. Cook for an additional 15 minutes, until the centers of the potatoes are soft and the edges are crisp.
8. Allow the chips to cool.
9. Cool and store in an airtight glass container for up to 7 days.

ADDITIONAL TOPPINGS

Boost the fall flavors and top with cinnamon and nutmeg. Or make them spicy with a bit of cayenne pepper, hot paprika, or everything blend from Trader Joe's.

MOROCCAN SPICED CHICKPEAS

MAKES 1 CUP

These Moroccan-inspired chickpeas—loaded with flavor, fun, and lots of anti-inflammatory spices and seasonings—can be eaten as a healthy snack or added to your favorite salads, soups or plant-based beauty bowls.

INGREDIENTS

- 1 15 ½ ounce can chickpeas, drained and rinsed
- 1 tablespoon grapeseed, olive, or avocado oil
- ¼ teaspoon ground cumin
- ¼ teaspoon ground ginger
- ¼ teaspoon ground cinnamon
- ¼ teaspoon ground chile powder
- Pinch of cayenne pepper or hot paprika
- ½ teaspoon sea salt

PREP

1. Preheat the oven to 400°F.
2. Dry the chickpeas by rolling them in a paper towel or a kitchen towel.
3. Combine the oil and the spices in a large bowl. Add the chickpeas and toss until evenly coated with the spice mixture.
4. Spread the chickpeas on a parchment-lined baking sheet.
5. Bake the chickpeas until golden and crunchy, about 25–35 minutes, stirring them occasionally.
6. Let the chickpeas cool completely.
7. Store in a glass airtight container. Spiced chickpeas will last for about two weeks. You can also freeze them for parties or use at another time. Simply thaw and reheat until hot and crisp.

RADIANT TIP

Mix and match spices by adding or deleting, or create your own blend.

BEYOND RADIANT
WARM APPLE CRISP

SERVES 4

If you love apples and indulging in an occasional sweet treat, then this is the perfect crisp for you. Great for the holidays, an intimate dinner party, or anytime you crave something delicious, satisfying, and pleasurable without refined sugar, dairy, or gluten.

INGREDIENTS

- 5 medium apples, thinly sliced (I prefer a blend of apples: red, pink ladies, and fuji)
- ½ lemon
- Ground cinnamon to taste
- 1 cup almond flour
- 3 tablespoons of coconut oil
- ½ cup crushed walnuts

PREP

1. Preheat the oven to 375°F.
2. Layer the apples on an 8 x 8 baking dish. Squeeze the lemon over the apples, evenly covering them with juice. Generously sprinkle the apples with cinnamon.
3. In a small bowl, combine the almond flour and coconut oil.
4. Sprinkle mixture over apples. Bake the crisp for 40 minutes, or until the apples are soft.
5. Serve warm. Or keep in the refrigerator and eat for breakfast the next day. Yum.

PUMPKIN PIE WITH HEALTHY COCONUT WHIPPED CREAM

SERVES 6

I grew up loving pumpkin pie, and still do. This healthy version lets you indulge in all the nutrient-dense pleasures of pumpkin without feeling weighed down by the refined sugars and processed dairy. Pumpkin is naturally high in vitamin A (skin- and immunity-boosting), potassium (cardiovascular supportive), and plant polyphenols, like lutein (eyesight protective). This pie is simple to make and super satisfying too.

INGREDIENTS

- 2 cups organic pumpkin puree
- 2 eggs
- ½ cup monk fruit
- 1 tablespoon pumpkin pie spice
- 1 teaspoon cinnamon
- ¼ teaspoon sea salt
- 1 cup full fat coconut milk, unsweetened

PREP

1. Preheat the oven to 350°F.
2. Lightly grease a glass pie dish with coconut oil.
3. Combine all ingredients in a bowl. Whisk until thoroughly combined.
4. Pour the mixture into the prepared pie dish.
5. Bake for 60 minutes, or until a toothpick comes out clean

HEALTHY COCONUT
WHIPPED CREAM

MAKES 1 CUP

You will love this easy-peasy, healthy version of coconut whipped cream. Give it a try and let me know how you like it.

INGREDIENTS

- 1 cup full fat coconut cream, unsweetened
- 1 teaspoon pure vanilla extract

PREP

1. Chill the can of coconut cream in the refrigerator overnight, up to 24 hours.
2. Place the chilled coconut cream in a mixing bowl with the vanilla and whip until fluffy.
3. Store the whipped coconut cream in a sealed container in the refrigerator.

MARLYN'S MATCHA BEAUTY BLISS BALLS

MAKES ABOUT 50 1 ½-INCH BLISS BALLS

Simple, nutrient-dense beauty treats to help you keep calm, fit, fueled, and satisfied for hours on end.

INGREDIENTS

- ¾ cup pitted dates (about 6 dates)
- 1 cup raw cashews
- 2 teaspoons matcha green tea powder
- 2 tablespoons coconut oil
- ¼ teaspoon cinnamon
- ¼ teaspoon vanilla bean powder
- ¼ teaspoon salt
- Shredded coconut for rolling

PREP

1. Add the dates and the cashews to a food processor or high-speed blender and pulse until the dates and cashews are coarsely ground.
2. Add the matcha powder, coconut oil, cinnamon, vanilla bean powder, and salt. Process for 2–3 minutes until the ingredients start to blend together. Scrape down sides as needed. The mixture should hold its shape when pinched between your fingers. Add a teaspoon or two of water if your mixture is dry.
3. Gently roll the dough into 1 ½-inch balls and roll again in shredded coconut (or other ingredients below).
4. Store in the refrigerator. Enjoy!

RADIANT TIP

Explore rolling your Bliss Balls in other tasty ingredients like cinnamon, raw cacao, hemp seeds, and/or a dash of sea salt, or try a combo of each. To boost brain power, consider adding in 1–1 ½ teaspoons of lion's mane. For extra beauty, add ½ teaspoon of pearl powder.

SPA-INSPIRED CHOCOLATE TREATS

MAKES ABOUT 50 1-INCH PIECES

These delicious, spa-inspired treats taste great while keeping your blood sugar balanced, your energy elevated, and your waistline trim. They're the perfect little rejuvenating bite when you need an afternoon lift, travel snack, or a simple pleasurable indulgence to keep your sexy goddess side going for hours on end. Enjoy!

INGREDIENTS

- 3 tablespoons coconut oil
- ¼ cup raw cacao powder
- ½ cup almonds, hazelnuts, or cashews, ground
- ¾ cup unsweetened shredded coconut

- Optional: ½–1 teaspoon pearl powder, ashwagandha, reishi, or lion's mane

PREP

1. Over low heat in a small saucepan, melt but do not simmer the honey and coconut oil in a saucepan.
2. Blend thoroughly and pour the warm mixture into a bowl.
3. Add the cacao, ground nuts, and coconut to the warm oil/honey mixture and thoroughly incorporate.
4. Pour the mixture onto a small baking sheet covered with parchment paper.
5. When cool to touch, form into a square.
6. Refrigerate until hardened. Break into bite-size servings.
7. Store in a glass container in your refrigerator or freezer.

Tip: A Magic Bullet works great when grinding the nuts

LEMON-GINGER ICED TEA
WITH FRESH MINT

MAKES 6 SERVINGS

Spruce up your day with a delicious cup of refreshing lemon-ginger iced tea. It's easy to make and good for you. In addition to the antioxidants in the green tea, it contains a dose of vitamin C from the citrus fruits and anti-inflammatory goodness from the ginger.

INGREDIENTS

- 1 cup blueberries, rinsed
- Water for the ice cube trays, plus 8 cups water, divided
- ⅓ cup coarsely chopped fresh ginger
- 6 green tea bags, or 3 teaspoons of matcha tea
- 2 lemons, juiced (about ½ cup)
- 1 orange, juiced (about ½ cup)
- Lemon slices
- Mint sprigs, for garnish

For a touch of sweetness, add manuka honey, lucama, or monk fruit

PREP

1. Six hours before serving the iced tea, place about 4 berries in each compartment of an ice cube tray. Fill the tray with water and freeze.
2. Place 2 cups of water and the ginger in a saucepan and bring to a boil.
3. Reduce heat and simmer over low heat for 5 minutes.
4. Remove the ginger water from heat and add the tea bags.
5. Let the mixture steep for at least 30 minutes and up to 1 hour.
6. Strain out solids.
7. In a pitcher, combine strained liquid with 6 cups of water and the lemon juice. Chill in the refrigerator.
8. To serve, place the ice cubes in a tall glass and pour iced tea over cubes.
9. Garnish with lemon slices and mint sprigs.

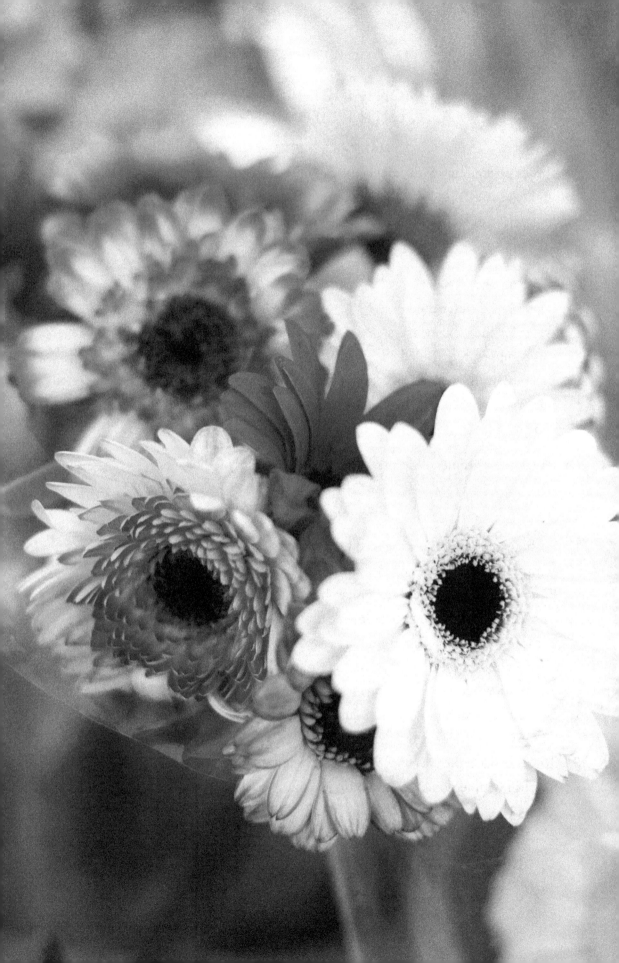

Chapter 11

CHECKING IN AND STAYING ON TRACK

I attribute my success to this:
I never gave or took any excuses.

— FLORENCE NIGHTINGALE

You've changed your diet and are eating differently now. You feel radiant and healthy. And yet you wonder, how do I stay on track for the long run?

It's easier than you think because you already have a system in place. And here is where you get to choose what works best for you. Set up a schedule of check-ins and celebrate those small milestones you've achieved along the way. All you really need to do is to recommit to your beautiful self each and every day.

Maybe you've learned to cook a new recipe, dropped a jean size, or are training for a 5K marathon. Or perhaps you've made it up that difficult hill you've been trying to climb for years. Better still, maybe your glucose levels or your A1c numbers have improved.

What has helped my clients and me stay on track is to include the transformational food cleanse once or twice and year and making sure we get our blood tests once a year. We have the power to remain mindful, to choose the food that nourishes us and the activities that serve us and others. This is our new lifestyle and not a quick-fix diet plan.

To help you thrive on your new path, here are tools to empower you as you travel, eat out, or attend that special event. Once you have the tools, there's no reason to live any other way than healthFULLY. And yes, you can cheat here and there. Sip your wine or vodka spritzer. Indulge in your favorite dessert, or delicious dark chocolate.

For those special treats, practice the Three-Bite Rule, and follow the tips below. You'll be satisfied and pleasurized, AND you'll experience lasting success without the guilt, bloat, and regret.

STAYING COMMITTED

HEALTHY TRAVEL

A big part of sustaining a healthy lifestyle is knowing how to handle travel and eating on the go. Whether you're traveling for business, work, or pleasure, to another state or country, rituals and routines will keep you going strong. Here are my first-class travel tips.

BEYOND RADIANT HEALTHY TRAVEL TIPS

Airports and hotels have become much more accustomed to supporting healthy lifestyles. Salads and meals that carry calorie counts and a clear list of ingredients are easily available.

But be aware:, hotels and airports are also there to sell you stuff—junk food, drinks, candy, crackers. Many airports and some hotels actually hire specific design teams to create layouts that promote the sale of food through enticing smells that lure you in and tempt you to part with your money. (Think baked cinnamon buns, pizza, and chocolate donuts.) Most of the time you would never think of buying that cinnamon bun with its thick layer of icing, but there it is right in front of you, with its sugary-buttery-cinnamony aroma appealing to your senses (especially if you have a bit of anxiety about flying or traveling).

By taking a proactive approach and sticking with fruit, nuts, salads, protein bars with whole-food ingredients, and proteins like chicken, shrimp, or hard-boiled eggs, you will vanquish your cravings and keep your hunger hormones in check.

BELOW ARE THE THINGS THAT HAVE HELPED ME,
AND MY CLIENTS, STAY ON TRACK:

- **Be Prepared:** When traveling on Airlines, **BYOS:** Bring Your Own Snacks.
- **Hotel:** Call ahead and ask the hotel to empty the mini fridge. If you like to make shakes, ask for a blender to be delivered to your room, or bring your own.
- **Swing by a grocery store** on the way to your hotel. Consider stocking up on bottled water, lemons, fresh fruit, avocado, almonds, carrot sticks, nut milk, and a jar of nut butter—all good options for breakfasts and healthy snacks.
- **Before you leave (or during your stay), Google "healthy restaurants"** in the area where you are traveling. Make a reservation if you're planning to eat out.

HEALTHY TRAVEL SNACKS TO PACK FOR YOUR TRIP

- **Bars:** Real ingredient bars with minimal ingredients, like Lärabars, RxBars, or others.
- **Nuts and nut butters:** Almonds, walnuts, cashews, macadamias, or mix your own. Individual nut butter packets are convenient and delicious when it comes to traveling. Pair with an apple, half of a banana, or another fruit of choice.
- **Gluten-free crackers:** Skinny Crisps, Jilz Crackers, and Mary's Gone Crackers are a few favorite varieties.
- **Fruit and veggies:** Whole or cut-up apples, pears, blueberries, baby carrots, jicama, cucumbers, Chinese pea pods, and celery are all easy for travel. Bring a few slices of lemon on your flight. Add them to hot water. Lemon water is great for hydration and for reducing jet lag.
- **Protein:** Tuna in individual pop-top cans, edamame, grilled shrimp, hard-boiled eggs, turkey roll-ups on lettuce or seaweed, and hummus are all simple choices that pack a lot of nourishment and protein staying power.
- **Herbal tea:** I'm a big fan of bringing a few packets of herbal tea on the plane. My favorites are Numi brand rooibos and rooibos chai and tulsi holy basil.

All are caffeine-free and support a calm nervous system. Other favorites are ginger and peppermint, which are wonderful for digestion.

- **Water:** Purchase a bottle or two. Look for natural spring water when possible. Stay hydrated to lessen jet lag and support enhanced cellular energy.

- **Let it flow:** Take along some fiber to avoid constipation that sometimes occurs during travel. Good choices are ground flaxseeds and chia seeds. Magnesium oxide tablets and pitted prunes can be helpful too. Pack some green powder in small baggies for the amount of days you are away.

- **Exercise:** Please don't skip the exercise. Pack exercise clothes. Go for a walk or to the hotel gym or pool. Or try dancing in your room to your favorite music.

A TOOLBOX OF TIPS FOR EATING OUT

LITTLE TIPS THAT YIELD BIG RESULTS

1. Ask the waiter **not** to bring bread to the table or fries with anything.
2. Avoid fried foods. When ordering fish, ask that it be broiled or sautéed. Kindly request that your fish be prepared with olive oil or real butter.
3. Order your vegetables to be steamed with a side of olive oil for dipping. Or, if you prefer a bit more flavor with your greens and veggies, ask that they be sautéed in olive oil, herbs, and garlic.
4. At lunch order salads with lean proteins. Local fish is always a good choice. Avoid buns, breads, and paninis. Use lettuce as a wrap instead of bread.
5. Ask for dressing on the side, or olive oil and lemon, if you wish. Avocado and sea salt are great additions for healthy fat and added flavor.
6. Get an extra vegetable and/or salad instead of bread or pasta.
7. Consider sharing an entree with a side of soup or salad.
8. Drink a glass of water just after you sit down at the table, or sip hot water with lemon with your meal.

GIRLS' NIGHT OUT, YOUR FIRST DATE, YOUR SON OR DAUGHTER'S WEDDING

There's no reason to blow all your good results when you're out for girls' night, on a date, or at another festive occasion. Make eating out a fun and playful adventure—a change from the ordinary. (My inner East Coast girl loves a fun foodie night out! How about you?) Choose wisely. Look for healthy fare and hip restaurants that use farm-fresh ingredients. And remember, you can always Google the restaurant before you leave your home or hotel room to look over the menu and get familiar with their selections and specials.

Italian Restaurant: Try your best to stay clear of the bread basket. Opt for a house green salad instead. Add olive oil, fresh lemon, and sea salt. Good fats equal a good brain boost. Have a bowl of vegetable or minestrone soup as a starter to curb appetite.

Instead of wheat pasta, choose gluten-free pasta or veggies like spinach, string beans, or grilled veggies. Ask to have your sauce of choice poured over the veggies instead of the pasta. You've lowered your carb load and your after-dinner glycemic load. Choose red meat sauce, veggie sauce with roasted eggplant, or red seafood sauce. Stay away from creamed sauces, which are high fat and loaded with dairy and butter. Fish and grilled veggies are a very good option. One of my favorite dishes is a simple grilled chicken breast with olive oil, garlic, and herbs.

Indian: Your best options are chicken tikka, chicken tandoori, or shrimp tandoori. Stay clear of creamed sauces like chicken tikka masala. Fresh curry sauces, made with coconut milk, are a better option. If you have rice, keep your serving to 1/2 cup. Plain basmati or vegetable basmati are good choices. Skip the naan. Opt for a few papadam, which are usually made with lentil flour instead of wheat.

Look for fresh veggie dishes made with cauliflower, spinach, or okra. My favorite is plain sag (sautéed spinach with fresh onions, garlic, and tomatoes.) Many Indian dishes are also made with cheese. Ask if your dish can be made without the cheese. A bit of beef or lamb can be nice. Pair them with grilled onions and peppers. Baingan bharta, made with eggplant, is a flavorful plant-based vegan dish loaded with immune-boosting onions, ginger, and garlic. Drink hot water and lemon to aid digestion. A small green salad can be nice as well.

When chosen properly, nutrient-rich dishes rooted in authentic Indian culture and cuisine make a wonderful flavor-rich meal infused with an abundance of healing herbs and spices that support well-being, gut-health, and immunity.

Thai: Thai restaurants often offer an array of seafood in addition to an abundance of vegetables. Clear broth soups or tom yum pair well with added seafood or chicken. Remember to keep your serving of rice to ½ cup. Brown rice is best, if available. Thai lettuce or rice paper wraps with fresh veggies are nice starters.

Choose white sauces over brown because white sauces usually have less sodium and no soy. Many brown sauces contain salt, soy, and some may even have MSG. If you are truly watching your weight and carbs, opt for steamed chicken, shrimp, seafood, and veggies. Order a side of peanut sauce and use it sparingly for a burst of flavor.

Chinese: Consider wonton soup minus the wontons. Opt for protein, veggies, and minimal brown or white rice. If you crave a stir-fry, choose the white sauces over brown. (Brown sauces are usually loaded with more sugar.) Skip the fried shrimp and fried beef because these usually are breaded and deep-fried. Steamed eggplant with a side of peanut sauce can be nice as well. And don't forget the greens. Chinese restaurants often have many wonderful greens available for sauté.

French: I congratulate you for entering a French restaurant, synonymous with copious amounts of bread, butter, and wine, not to mention creamy sauces. Stick with a simple piece of broiled fish or a nice piece of chicken with herbs. Ask if you can have your food made with olive oil instead of butter. French restaurants are known for their lovely endive salads. Order one. Bitter greens and herbs are cleansing to the liver.

Steak House: Are you a woman who loves a good steak? I say go for it! Choose leaner cuts like filets or rib eyes and tenderloins. Choose a higher-quality steak house when possible to know you are getting a good product with little to no hormones. Grass-fed beef is best, of course. Most steak houses have lots of good veggies on their menu too. Order up some sides like grilled asparagus, sautéed spinach, roasted sweet potatoes, grilled mushrooms, and a nice house salad. Request that your food be prepared in olive oil over butter.

Sushi: Lots of good options here. Choose fresh sashimi over sushi. If you want rice, keep your serving size to ½ cup, and preferably brown rice if available. That translates to four pieces of sushi or two hand or cut rolls. Stay clear of the fried stuff and lots of sauces. Order miso soup, salad, or steamed edamame for your appetizer. Most sushi places have a nice ginger or miso dressing. Order it on the side so you can control how much you put on. Use sparingly. You can also ask for olive oil, fresh lemon, and sea salt for your salad. Order a great big salad and a few sides of sashimi and make your own sashimi salad. Top with avocado for extra flavor and a brain health boost. Ginger and wasabi are very nice meal enhancers and cleanse the palate. If you like hand rolls, consider ordering hand rolls with chopped albacore or yellowtail and no rice. (Or easy rice—that's less rice in Los Angeles talk.) Add in sliced avocado and cucumber for an extra veggie boost. Top with a little wasabi and ask for tamari sauce, or bring your own. Don't laugh; many of my clients have been known to do that. Some of my clients who frequent neighborhood sushi restaurants even leave their bottle there with the chef behind the counter.

Listen Up! Okay, I know you women. I'm one of you. We don't like to make a fuss, bring attention to ourselves, or have our friends think we're on some crazy diet plan. So, let's reframe our thinking. This is *our* health, and if we choose to avoid calling attention to ourselves, we can simply ask the waiter to kindly come over. We can talk softly to him as our colleagues or friends are chatting along and downing their drinks. Most likely no one will be paying attention and we'll feel better when eating our meals that were prepared with health and flavor in mind.

Special Note: If you're cleansing, I'd highly consider avoiding the alcohol and order sparkling water or Perrier with lime. And if you really want that shot of booze, have a clean cocktail minus any mixtures or sugary add-ons. Vodka or tequila with lots of fresh lime makes an especially nice and refreshing drink. And it's gluten-free and keto-approved too.

RADIANT TIP

HOT LEMON WATER

In between meals, or at the end of the meal, consider sipping hot water with lemon. Lemon water is a great palate cleanser and digestive aid.

THE THREE-BITE RULE

This is the golden rule I use and teach to my clients. This allows us to indulge without feeling deprived and blowing all our hard work. The rule is simple: You can take three bites of anything you love, if you must, but the fourth bite brings diminishing returns. If you are at a dinner party or out with your friends and you don't want to seem rude or are asked to share a slice of birthday cake, have three bites, enjoy them, and then stop. If having three bites triggers you to want more and you're unable to put your fork down until you finish the whole piece, then consider this particular food a red light food and stop before you start. Some of us especially get triggered by sugar. So know yourself and instill discipline where you need it.

DIANA'S WELLNESS JOURNEY

Down Twenty Pounds, Healthier Habits, and a Renewed Sense of Joy and Adventure for Life!

Diana walked into our last few coaching sessions with a skip in her step, a smile on her face, and an attitude that said, YES, I can! Her confidence had grown during our six months working together. She dropped twenty pounds. She appeared to be more in flow with life: surrendering to the things that were out of her control and taking healthy consistent action steps on the things that she could control like what she ate and how she exercised, and developing a positive, open, mindset.

She had a fresh new spirit about her too. I saw it immediately when she walked into my office dressed in soft, feminine clothes, colorful cashmere sweaters, pointy-toed pumps, slimming jeans, playful T-shirts, and fitted dresses. A gorgeous woman from the start, Diana, with her medium-brown bob, gracious ways, and incredible smarts, was experiencing an inner shift, which was coming through loud and clear in her positive new attitude, joyful disposition, and beaming healthy radiance. Honestly, it was miraculous to witness.

In recapping our time together, I asked Diana to name the things that supported her most in stepping toward fifty with more confidence and joy. I also asked her to share helpful tips that others may benefit from when they start their own wellness journey.

Here's what she shared:

"Without a doubt, changing my mindset and implementing new, healthier habits has been number one in contributing to my overall success. My top tips for anyone ready to begin their own wellness journey are the following."

HEALTHY HABITS + CONSISTENCY = SUCCESS

1. Keep choosing the good/healthy.
2. Learn how to live in the gray.There are a lot of wellness tools available. Find the tools that fit and work for you.
3. We are all different and need different things. Customize your tools.
4. Meditate, for at least three minutes a day.
5. Create structure. Structure helped set me up for sustainable success!

WHAT'S MY WHY?

"If veering off the path, ask yourself, 'What's my WHY? Why am I doing this in the first place?' Honestly, this has REALLY helped me, especially on Valentine's Day when I went off path with a chocolate binge. There were See's Candies everywhere! I indulged. Which was fine for a day or two. Then it was way too much and I began asking myself, 'What's going on here, Diana?' I looked back at when I was last doing well. I remembered a few weeks before Valentine's Day, I got the flu and I started craving sugar.

"Without this journey, my old all or nothing thinking would have taken me down a rabbit hole and right back to my unhealthy ways of eating. This time, I stopped, paused, and reminded myself to stick to it. I treated myself with kindness, recognized I'm human, used the ACE formula, and elevated my chocolate to a healthier version (which I only now have on occasion) and got back on track. That was a HUGE win and a new way of doing things for me.

MINDSET

"I had to shed the diet mentality I grew up with. I realized how much it was shaping my decisions. When we went on vacation, food and calories 'didn't count.' Those vacation calories were freebies. My parents would eat whatever they wanted, and as soon as we got home, they were back on their diet. I adopted similar views, until I realized they were not supporting my current wants, goals, and desires in life, at all."

MAKE THINGS AN ADVENTURE!

1. Try new restaurants: I enjoyed all the healthy new restaurants I experienced on my six-month wellness journey. It's been wonderful to get out of my comfort zone and try fun new foods.

2. Plow through resistance: When I'm faced with things I resist wanting to do, I try to make an adventure out of it. Like the time I had to drive really far to my kids' sports tournament by myself. Instead of dreading it, I made it fun. I listened to great music on the drive, stopped at my favorite coffee place, and even tried a healthy restaurant I had read about months ago. I ended up loving every minute!

"This wellness journey has been one heck of a ride, and I'm beyond excited to take the next steps in my life, and keep the good stuff going.

I know this new path will be an ever-blossoming adventure, and I will do all that I can to embrace it with love, joy, commitment. and an open heart. Fifty, here I come!"

LIFE HAPPENS AND THEN WE HEAL

Let's face it, in life our bodies and their precious parts can wear down, become damaged, need a lift, or, on occasion, need to be removed completely. If, or when, you opt for surgery, here are a few tips to bring with you into the clinic or hospital, feeling strong and ready to heal on the other end.

SURGERY AND SCAR TISSUE

With surgery, it's possible to develop scar tissue. This is where the tissue around the surgery site gets hard. Scar tissue can sometimes be painful as well. To help break down scar tissue, consider taking proteolytic enzymes about a week or so after the surgery (with your doctor's approval). Think of these guys as little Pac-Men that are eating up the scar tissue. Take these enzymes between meals, as they work better on an empty stomach.

Other supplements that help heal surgery scars and inflammation are:
- Vitamin C (I prefer buffered)
- Zinc
- VitD
- Omega 3
- Arnica

Again, consult with your doctor before taking any supplements before or after surgery.

Foods that have been researched to support healing:
- Pineapple (contains bromelain)
- Papaya (contains papain enzymes)

RADIANT TIP

STOCK YOUR PANTRY BEFORE SURGERY

Before you go in for a surgical procedure that will require recovery time in bed, take time to prepare your body and your cupboard. After your procedure, you want to have what you need to feel comforted and heal better. I recommend stocking your fridge and pantry with healing foods like soups (homemade or purchased), bone broth, fresh green and vegetable juices, fruits packed with vitamin C like grapefruit (avoid if on blood thinners), berries, and oranges. Protein helps your body heal after a trauma. If you eat meat, consider purchasing an organic rotisserie chicken from your local market, or prepare a pot of chicken soup. Perhaps you can ask a friend to make a fresh pot of soup for you. Remember to follow your doctor's recommendations. Depending upon your needs, a well-stocked fridge and pantry will allow you extra time to rest and recoup.

RADIANT TIP

POSITIVE VISUALIZATION

In 2001, I read a phenomenal book called *Women's Bodies, Women's Wisdom* by Dr. Christiane Northrup. In it, Dr. Northrup shares a beautiful way to enter into any surgical procedure. She suggests that you ask your anesthesiologist and/or surgeon to recite an affirmation as you are going under anesthesia. The affirmation can be written out on a card, if you wish, and can sound something like this: "This procedure will be extremely effective and smooth and you will heal beautifully and quickly." You can tweak those words as you see fit.

The idea behind the practice is that we are planting powerful messages into the brain so that we can heal with grace and positivity. I've used this practice personally and it has helped me during various surgeries and procedures I've had over the years. It also made me feel that the doctors and surgeons on my team were rooting for my healing.

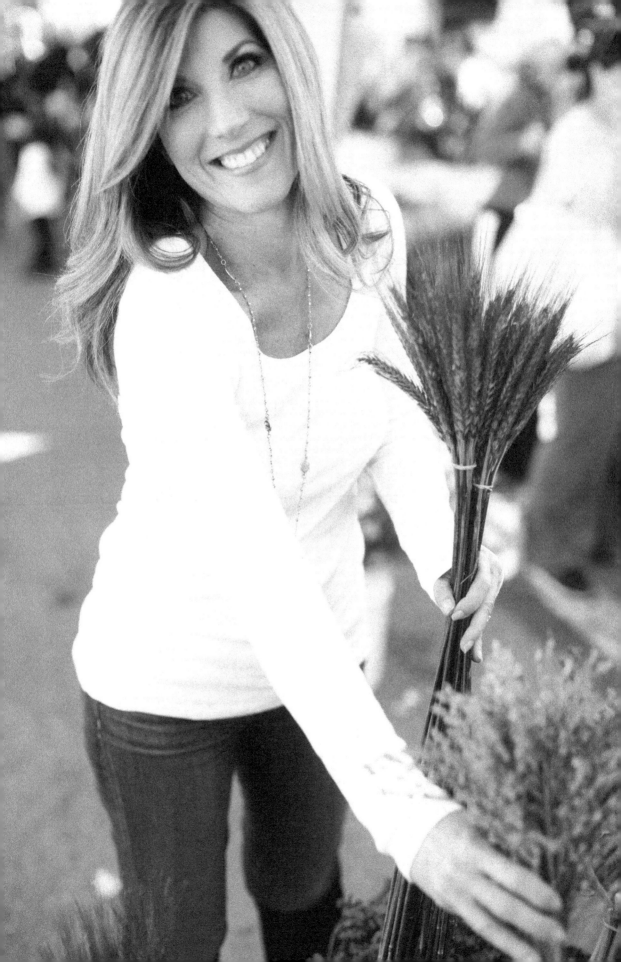

Chapter 12

LIVE, LOVE, RADIATE!

Sweet friend, it's been beautiful to share this journey with you. Know that I am here cheering you on, always. I believe in you. I trust in you. I have faith in you. As a closing gift, I'm sharing pieces of my heart—with love. These are notes I wrote, lessons I learned, pain I healed, love I found. Many are revelations from the sacred moments I've experienced with clients. May they bring you peace, comfort, an uplift, inspiration, and joy on your ever-blossoming path. You are not alone.

WAKING UP AT MIDLIFE

Live your most authentic life.
Give yourself permission to go after what you want.
To have what you want.
Create the history you desire.
Trust the process and believe in you.
Write the book you want to read.
Let go of the shame. Anger. Frustration.
Do stuff you've never done before.
You get to choose what to think. Choose wisely.
Have a daily practice. Rituals.

Have a routine in place. Healthy habits.

Tenacity is a muscle. Build the muscle.

Keep the faith.

Keep showing up. You will get there.

You can do whatever you set your mind to.

Make a difference.

Own your success.

Live from a place of empowerment.

Give yourself permission.

Practice self-love.

Gratitude.

Lose the doubt.

Challenge the beliefs.

It's all an inside job.

Stand in it and own it.

Embody all your parts.

Own your power. Live from Love.

No comparing yourself.

Create prosperity.

Choose consciously.

Celebrate it all. It's an AWAKENING.

LET YOUR INNER GODDESS SHINE!

Your Inner Goddess is your inner light. She's the one who banishes all the shoulds and guilt imposed on you. She's one smart cookie, and she deserves to have a voice and to be listened to. She is your higher power, your intuition, your authentic truth. Own her. Give her permission to show up, speak, and shine.

We've been taught to be good girls, people pleasers, and selfless givers, sometimes so much so we forget ourselves, beat ourselves up, and judge ourselves fiercely.

How can we shine more and be our most radiant selves if all the parts of us are not allowed to be seen or heard? Give your Inner Goddess a voice. Chances are, she has something incredibly valuable to say.

SPIRITUALITY IN MIDLIFE

Find meaning and purpose.

If raising kids was a big part of your time and attention, and that period of your life has passed, honor it, celebrate it, and fill that void.

You are the wise woman, the wisdom keeper. Share your wisdom.

Connect to something bigger! Be of service. Give.

As things change, align with a purpose. Consider joining or starting a Wise Women's Circle, or join an organization (online or off) that feeds your soul. Someone special is waiting to meet you. In community we have the opportunity to connect, heal, grow, and uplift ourselves and each other. The time is now.

GETTING NEWER EVERY DAY

Instead of aging, think of yourself as getting newer every day. The path toward feeling newer enables you to follow your inner compass of joy. Your inner compass of joy gets activated when you are doing what excites you and what gives you purpose. First, the impulse (the spark), and then we take action.

In this way, the process of shifting to what excites you (instead of dwelling on what brings you down) becomes completely self-rewarding. It's *the thing* that can take you from good to great. From feeling down, depressed or anxious to feeling alive. We can become turned on by our inner impulse to create.

For example, after years of feeling sad and going through challenging times, the desire to write this book came from an internal spark. I sat down, dug in, and got real on paper. The more I wrote, the more it activated me and gave me purpose. The internal joy, the incredible pleasure, and the hope that my years of study, nutritional knowledge, experience, and life wisdom would make their way into the world to serve others became the juice that kept me going each day, the juice that still lights me up and turns me on!

There's joy in creating. There's life force too. The more you say yes to what excites you, the more you get turned on. As you continue on the path of life, stay curious. Live from a place of wonder, joy, and excitement. There's magic in the newness of each day.

50 TIPS FOR TURNING 50, 60 & BEYOND

Shortly after I turned fifty, I wrote this piece for Maria Shriver's blog, "Architects of Change."

There are many great tips for us all whether we're stepping into fifty, sixty, seventy, or beyond!

Turning fifty! For me there was a lot of excitement about this new milestone and a lot of uncertainty too. I had been through so much these last many years. Some good, some not so good. As I approached my big day, I asked myself, "What would the next decade bring?" And more importantly, "What did I want?" I spent the months leading up to this special day reflecting on what had supported me, elevated me, and strengthened me (inside and out) and celebrated with pride that I was feeling better at fifty than I did at thirty. I looked at the areas and the changes that had the greatest impact on my body, mind, and spirit. These included; food, fitness, finance, friends, family, and career. I recalled that in my younger years, I spent days hanging out with women who drained my energy, worked at unfulfilling jobs, avoided dealing with unpleasant financial statements, shopped to fill a void, and ate sugar to soothe my soul. This led to low energy, low confidence, low self-esteem, low bank accounts, health challenges, and a feeling of emptiness. Looking at where I am now, I relish the newfound confidence and beauty that I feel. Instead of running from my fiftieth birthday, I decided to embrace it. I invited all my heart-based soul-sister girlfriends to gather around and celebrate with me. The day was filled with pure joy. During my dessert toast, I thanked everyone for coming and reflected in gratitude on my purpose-driven fulfilling nutrition career, my strong health-based eating plan, my fit body, and my loving family and friends. It was one of the happiest days of my life!

What I know for sure is that it's the simple steps and the daily actions we take each day that create the radiant, vibrant body and life we crave.

Below are simple steps that have worked for me and the many people I serve. This list highlights the top tips that I've learned from working at top-rated integrative medical centers, attending nutrition conferences, taking mindfulness classes, reading books, supporting clients, and real life living. They are science-based, heart-based, and health-based. Take your power back, turn the clock around, and rediscover that sexy, vibrant, energetic you.

1. Drink green juice.
2. Take a hike in nature.
3. Have lunch with an old friend.
4. Have lunch with a new friend.
5. Eat some greens.
6. Watch a funny movie.
7. Drink water with lemon.
8. Smile at a stranger.
9. Nix the artificial sweeteners.
10. Stop and smell the roses.
11. Add a green powder to your morning.
12. Call a childhood friend and reminisce about the fun times growing up.
13. Find an exercise routine you love. DO IT!
14. Eat at a healthy restaurant.
15. Add a probiotic to your day.
16. Sit in a lobby of a luxury hotel and enjoy the beauty.
17. Make dinner for a friend.
18. Purchase a pretty new sweater that makes your eyes pop!
19. Eat snacks and meals made up of healthy fat, fiber, and protein.
20. Add some color to your wardrobe.
21. Eat every 3–4 hours to keep your blood sugar balanced.
22. Meditate.
23. Drink holy basil tea because it's hormone balancing and calming.
24. Live in gratitude.
25. Declutter a drawer, room, or your closet.
26. Eat the rainbow.

27. BREATHE.

28. Hang out with some happy kids.

29. Walk barefoot in the grass.

30. Dance.

31. Drink a superfood smoothie for breakfast. Add some greens for an extra boost.

32. Aim for 6–8 hours of sleep.

33. Make a new healthy dish.

34. SLOW down! Chew your food.

35. Take a new route to work. Mix it up. Enjoy the scenery.

36. Connect with extraordinary people, movers and shakers, and wise women.

37. Tell your loved ones you love them.

38. Look in the mirror and tell yourself, "I love you!" (Sometimes harder to do than it sounds! ;-))

39. Pet a dog.

40. Repeat #30.

41. Get your teeth cleaned.

42. Get a mammogram, Pap smear, colonoscopy, and skin check. You will feel better knowing you did.

43. Travel to a new and exciting destination. Even if it's local.

44. Get your financial life in order including wills, estate planning, and daily living.

45. Know where important papers and documents are.

46. Eat breakfast. Add in some protein and healthy fat for satiety and prolonged energy.

47. Add more plant foods to your day.

48. Reduce caffeine intake.

49. Up your water consumption. Drink half your weight in ounces daily.

50. Enjoy the journey!

KEEP PRACTICING

Most of us have experienced how easy it can be to get lost in the busyness of our lives where sometimes even our good nutrition intentions and self-care habits can get lost, if we're not paying attention. This is especially true during the holiday season, life transitions, or an unexpected challenging life event.

My intention for you is to keep practicing. I made the list below as a reminder of what's always available. Consider taking a picture of the list and keeping it with you. Use it as a reminder to know that you have the power to slow down and keep the good stuff going—even through life's ups and downs, or any messy moments.

I AM CHOOSING

To slow down and be present.

To nourish my body, mind, and spirit daily.

To show up with love, even when it's uncomfortable.

To stop playing small.

To live a big life, even when it's messy.

To drop perfectionism.

To forgive myself, and others.

To trust more.

To have more gratitude.

To live a simpler life, and only buy the things I truly need.

To live in joy.

To invite joy in.

To let go of the people, places, things that no longer serve me—and to bless them all for the lessons they have taught me.

To show up every day believing in myself and my ability to create my life.

18 HEALTHY HABITS FOR EVERY WOMAN

1. Each body is unique. Listen to yours.
2. Speak your truth.
3. Spend time in nature.
4. Become your own health advocate. Seek a second or third opinion, if needed.
5. Detox—including toxic friends, toxic foods, and toxic emotions. They can all contribute to ill health.
6. Learn to cook. Even if it's one meal. You will feel proud.
7. Become a food detective. Read labels.
8. Never be afraid to step into your power. It's inside waiting to be unleashed.
9. Invite joy IN!
10. Live with passion and purpose. Do things you love to do.
11. Love your body and your life.
12. Dance, stretch, and move daily. A great way to keep your body strong.
13. Eat the rainbow. Good for your heart and your health.
14. Seek pleasure. It's yours for the taking.
15. Look for the blessings. They are all around you.
16. Add some fresh veggies to your day. Your skin will thank you.
17. Surround yourself with amazing women.
18. Let go and enjoy the journey.

ENDINGS

We play
We pause
We practice
We preach
We lose
We love
We shatter
We teach
And one day it ends
We strive to hold on

We grip

We latch

We clutch

Especially to the pleasure

Because these things define us

They shape us

They breathe new life into us

We laugh

We cry

We tussle

We tug

And one day it ends

Only to feel the pain

The pain is there to teach us

A reminder of what was

A glimpse of what's to come

All endings lead to new beginnings

Embrace them

Love them

Learn from them

Endings bring their sadness

Their joy

Their despair

Their reflections

Whatever the ending

Be fully in it

For without your presence

You will never know

All the life you just lived

And all the love that you are.

L.O.V.E.

Love is Love.

Love doesn't live in ego.

Love looks into another's eyes even when it's hard and talks about the tough stuff.

Love hugs, love hugs deeply, especially during the more challenging moments.

Love holds the other closely and says, "I'm here for you, as I can see you might be going through a tough time."

Love asks, "How can I help?"

Love shows up even when it wants to run.

Love remembers it is love and it loves, no matter what.

Love leads.

Love looks at their partner's eyes and asks, "What's going on?" and says "I'm here, come closer, I love you."

Love understands that maybe, just maybe, things can become difficult at times or uncomfortable because of life's circumstances or a moment that is hard, or a humanness that prevails out of angst, and love still shows up without ego and with a hug or a kiss or a song that says, I may not like this but I love you and I'm here.

Love sets the table for breakfast even when it doesn't want to.

Love is Love is Love.

There is only Love. Everything else is ego, judgment, reasoning, tension, stress, old wounds, new wounds, petty crap, old stories, childhood upsets—all disguised as Love.

Love is a friend, a lover, a partner—through thick and thin and all the good and all the yucky stuff too.

Love shows up as a heartfelt cheerleader even when times are tough and uncomfortable.

Love is Love.

Love is Love is Love. Nothing else but love.

May your days be filled with health, healing, and happiness.
Big Love. oxoxo

THE END/THE BEGINNING

ACKNOWLEDGEMENTS

To Joy: Editor, friend, and chief muse. WOW. WOW. WOW. I am forever grateful to Jill for connecting us. You listened to my vision and helped me bring it to life. More than your incredible editing and writing skills you have been a dear friend and listening ear as I shed, transformed, and morphed into a new version of myself. Writing a book is no easy feat. There were times I wanted to quit, pull my hair out, and jump off a cliff. You were there every step of the way encouraging me, listening to me and helping me to remember "My WHY!" Thank you for the gift of creating magic together. I loved our journey and look forward to the next one.

To Tim, Raquel, and Christine: Thank you for your talented and extraordinary interior graphic design, copyediting, and Public Relation skills. What a true blessing to have a wonderful "A-team" by my side.

To the Physicians, Healers, and Mentors — David Allen, M.D., Drew Francis, OMD, L.Ac, Farshad Rahbar, M.D., Harry Saperstein, M.D., Rachel Bar, Psy.D. LMFT and Carrie Tanenbaum, L.Ac: You taught me what it was to be a leader. You mirrored back how to help others transform their lives in body, mind and spirit. You inspire, educate, empower and enlighten me. You are the masters, mentors, and the incredible healers I've learned from through the years. Thank you.

To my Clients: I would never be where I am today without YOU. You hired me to teach you, though in return you have taught me so much more. Through serving you, you reflected back to me what is possible, what it is to be human. I am incredibly grateful for your honesty, heartfelt reflections, and love. It's been quite a blessing to watch you transform into the greatest versions of yourselves.

To my Business and Life Coaches: Michelle Baumen, Carolyn Freyer-Jones, Carey Peters, Stacey Morgenstern, and Liz Goldman. A huge THANK YOU from the bottom of my heart for guiding me, coaching me, and helping to see my gifts and my authentic self. Thank you for mirroring back to me that life is full of possibility, joy, and magic. You helped me grow in so many ways. Deep bow.

To the Movers, Shakers, and Rule Breakers: Oprah Winfrey, Maria Shriver, Michelle Obama, Diana Ross, Stevie Nicks, Rabbi Naomi Levy, Elizabeth Gilbert, Jean Chatsky, Bobbi Brown, Brené Brown, Danielle LaPorte, Marie Forleo, Jen Sincero, and Janet Mock. Thank you for inspiring me through the years. Thank you for leading the way, paving the path, and making it "cool" for creative, smart, entrepreneurial, bada$$, go-get-em women to shine their lights bright and be ALL of ourselves.

To my core Soul Sister Circle: Brenda, Gayle, Abby, Carrie, Joyce, Holli, Romy, Stacey, Stacy, Lori, Renee, and Andie: You are the wind beneath my wings. You are the light, love, kindness, and divine femine energy that has moved with me through each and every obstacle and over every mountain. I love you always.

To my Goddess Family: Barrie, Joyce, Aunt Carol, Jill, and Lynda. You are my "peeps." Thank you for being there when I needed to talk. Thank you for your love, light, laughter, friendship, and tried-and-true ways of caring and support. Life would never be the same without you. Forever grateful. I love you. Jill: a special thank you to you for designing the magnificent cover of this book. I love that it is wrapped in love and co-created by you.

Brad: Brother, friend, counsel. Through thick and thin, I am lucky to have your friendship and kind and loving support, always. Thank you for all the encouragement and financial advice, too. I love watching you grow (these last few years especially) and become the greatest version of yourself.

Dad and Sheila: You are my everything. Friends, family, counsel, quarantine netflix movie advisors, and greatest audience. Thank you for the countless conversations through the years. Thank you for the love, light, insights, and incredible teachings. The presence of your loving spirit has been one of the greatest blessings and gifts a daughter could ever ask for. I love you forever.

Mom: I miss you everyday. I know you are watching over me and have especially been with me through the journey of writing this book. I feel your presence every time a Monarch butterfly is near. Thank you for your guidance, love, support, cheerleading, and for teaching me how to dress with style. I love you

Doug: Thank you for coming into my life. Thank you for the love, laughter, fun, friendship, kindness, generosity, incredible support, massive growth and deep connection. This book would never have become what it has without you. I love you.

Ed: Together we made two beautiful boys. They are lucky to call you dad. Thank you for believing in my talents and inspiring me to "keep going" even when I wanted to give up. I especially appreciate that no matter what you and I were going through, you always reflected back to me to stay on path. I am grateful for all you have done to support my life, career and coaching journey, and I am proud of the ways we have grown. I love you for all of it.

Daniel and Josh: You are my light, love and greatest teachers. It's an honor to be your mom. You are both strong, independent, smart, caring and very "cool" young men. I love and miss the early years of raising you and am incredibly proud of the kind souls you turned out to be. My wish for you is that you continue to follow your heart and your dreams. And while you're making your mark and your millions, don't forget to call your mother. I love you, always.

To little Marlyn, young adult Marlyn and now Marlyn: You are one heck of a strong woman. Yes, you got knocked down a few times (maybe a lot of times), and you ALWAYS moved forward, taking the lessons from each and every event and allowing them to be integrated within you to make you stronger and wiser. What I appreciate about you more than anything is that you never let your heart close. Keep going girl, we're just getting started.

To the Universe: Thank you for co-creating this book with me. Thank you for my life and everything in it. You are magic.

To my higher power, intuition, and guiding force: I wake up each morning in gratitude knowing I am never alone. I am always supported knowing that you have my back. You are a strong and powerful presence in my life, Thank you for guiding me, protecting me, healing me and showing me my higher path.

ADAPTOGENS

GLOSSARY

Astragalus: Astragalus, high in flavonoids, is one of the most widely used tonics in Chinese medicine to promote *chi* or life force energy. Research indicates astragulus can help with immunity, longevity, lowering inflammation, oxidative stress, neurodegeneration, and brain health. It also has been studied to show positive anti-tumor effects.

Ashwangandha: This rejuvenating herb soothes anxiety, relieves stress, improves sleep, aids adrenal and thyroid health, and contributes to virility. Ashwagandha is said to give strength and stamina and bring calm.

Bacopa: Bacopa has been used for thousands of years by Ayurveda physicians to promote healthy brain function. Bacopa, also known as a nootropic, has been studied to improve concentration, focus, mood, reduce inflammation in the brain, improve intellect and memory, and support the central nervous system.

Chaga: A nutrient-dense mushroom that usually grows on a birch tree, chaga supports the aging process, promotes longevity, fights inflammation, and prevents the onset of degenerative diseases. Chaga is a rich source of superoxide dismutase, a powerful antioxidant, which has been studied to prevent damage to DNA. It has strong antiviral properties, boosts immunity, and balances blood sugar. Chaga also supports glowing skin, eyes, and hair.

Cordyceps: Cordyceps may support oxygenation of the body, mental power, endurance, sexual energy, muscle tone, and immunity.

He Shou Wu: This powerful herb may help improve stamina, enhance immunity, bring calm, and nourish the blood. It is also known to support hair, skin, and libido.

Lion's Mane: Lion's mane is a medicinal mushroom known to have therapeutic properties that promote nerve and brain health, specifically focus, enhanced concentration, cognitive impairment, and memory.

Maca: Maca is a nutrient powerhouse root native to Peru. It is traditionally used as an aphrodisiac and to support a healthy libido and sexual health. Maca may also help to improve energy, balance hormones, enhance sex drive, and boost memory. Many integrative medicine doctors and licensed acupuncturists support the health benefits of maca, though more research and human clinical trials are needed.

Matcha: I call matcha the Bentley of green teas. Matcha is made from the whole tea leaf and ground into a powder, allowing all the powerful constituents to go to work and support emotional and physical well-being. Matcha is known to help calm anxiety, boost metabolism, and cleanse the blood. It's super high in antioxidants, chlorophyll, and rich in L-theanine (which is calming). Studies show it supports breast health as well.

Mucuna Pruriens: Mucuna pruriens is a bean (aka the velvet bean) widely used in Ayurvedic medicine to help boost dopamine levels. Higher levels of dopamine have been linked to sound sleep and an expanded sense of well-being. Mucuna pruriens may help enhance brain function, elevate mood, soothe the nervous system, and support overall well-being.

Pearl Powder: Pearl is a revered longevity food that has been used for centuries by Taoist herbalists to support one's inner and outer radiance. It is an excellent source of minerals, including calcium, zinc, iron, selenium, and amino acids. Pearl has strong antioxidant and anti-inflammatory properties and helps to support the body's natural collagen production, promotes even and clear skin, strengthens bones, supports the nervous system, and promotes healthy sleep cycles.

Reishi: Reishi mushroom may help strengthen the immune system, support stress relief, and reduce systemic inflammation. Reishi has been a staple in Chinese medicine for over 2,000 years. It has a long history of promoting health and longevity. Reishi is a powerful antioxidant, which has been studied to neutralize free radicals and boost liver cell regeneration.

Shatavari: This amazing female rejuvenating herb is known in Ayurveda, the traditional system of medicine in India, as the Queen of herbs because it promotes love and devotion and helps boost vitality. It is commonly used to support menopause and female reproductive symptoms, longevity, immunity, and mental function. Shatavari is derived from the asparagus family and is high in phytochemicals, flavonoids, antioxidants, and trace minerals.

Schisandra Berry: This little red berry, grown in China and Russia, is known in Chinese medicine as the herb that does it all. High in antioxidants, polyphenols and vitamin C and E, schisandra is touted as a beautifying herb that helps purify the blood, support healthy libido, enhance memory and learning, and illuminate the skin by helping it to retain moisture and a youthful glow.

RESOURCES

SOME OF MY FAVORITES

ADAPTOGENS

Jing Herbs: jingherbs.com

Moon Juice: moonjuice.com

Sun Potion: sunpotion.com

Banyan Botanicals: banyanbotanicals.com

Four Sigmatic: us.foursigmatic.com

Navitas: navitasorganics.com

OM Mushrooms: ommushrooms.com

Feel Good Organics – Alma: fgorganics.com

NATURAL BEAUTY AND SKINCARE

The Detox Market: thedetoxmarket.com

CAP Beauty: capbeauty.com

Beauty Counter: beautycounter.com

Epicuren: epicuren.com

E.O.: eoproducts.com

FOODS I LOVE

GLUTEN-FREE BREAD

Breadblok: breadblok.com

Grindstone Bakery: grindstonebakery.com

PROTEIN POWDER

Epic Protein: sproutliving.com

Evolution_18 Collagen: evolution18.com

Moon Juice: moonjuice.com

Sun Warrior: sunwarrior.com

NUTS AND SEEDS

Go Raw: goraw.com

Trader Joe's: traderjoes.com

Ground Up Nut Butter: grounduppdx.com

Bob's Red Mill: bobsredmill.com

Spectrum (flaxseed): spectrumorganics.com

Health From the Sun (flaxseed): healthfromthesun.com

ORGANIC COFFEE

Stumptown: stumptowncoffee.com

Trader Joe's: traderjoes.com

Intelligentsia: intelligentsiacoffee.com

Canyon Coffee: canyoncoffee.com

OLIVE OIL

Melchiorri

TAHINI

Trader Joe's: amazon.com/Trader-Joes-Organic-Tahini-Butter

Seed + Mill: seedandmill.com

TEAS

Numi: numitea.com

DO Matcha: domatcha.com

Matcha Love: matchalove.com

Cap Beauty's The Matcha: capbeauty.com

CHOCOLATE AND CACAO

Pascha: paschachocolate.com

Hu: hukitchen.com

Navitas: navitasorganics.com

SPICES

Simply Spice: simplyorganic.com

WATER FILTER

Berkey: berkeyfilters.com

ORGANIC AND NATURAL
SEXUAL WELLNESS PRODUCTS

Good Clean Love: goodcleanlove.com

SUPPLEMENTS

If you are interested in learning more about professional grade supplements or the "Beyond Radiant Cleanse & Wellness Bundles," check out my online supplement store on Wellevate.

Wellevate: https://wellevate.me/marlyn-diaz

LET'S STAY CONNECTED!

www.marlynwellness.com

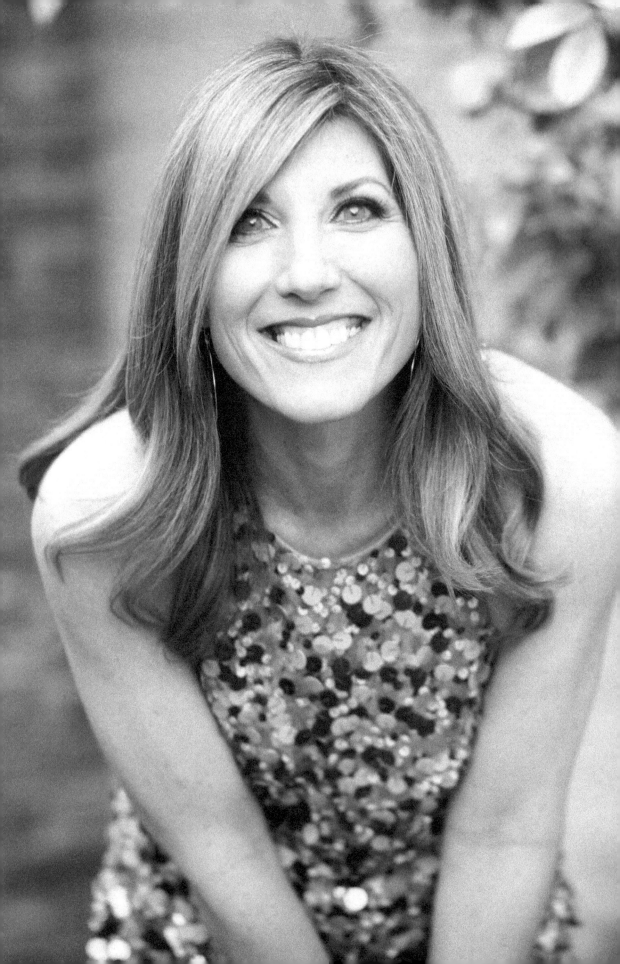

ABOUT THE AUTHOR

Marlyn Diaz is a leading Los Angeles–based Certified Nutritionist, Lifestyle Educator, and Wellness Coach specializing in weight management and rejuvenation for women and men. Marlyn received her BSc in Nutrition from Drexel University in Philadelphia and Certified Lifestyle Educator certification from Metagenics. She has been working in the food and nutrition industry for over twenty-five years. Marlyn delivers innovative solutions, unique accountability methods, simple tools, and science-based strategies that allow her clients to thrive in both their personal and professional lives while also delivering long-lasting weight loss and extraordinary health.

For fourteen years, Marlyn Diaz has contributed regularly to health-focused websites and magazines including MariaShriver.com, YouBeauty.com, and Mind Body Green. She was the Consulting Nutritionist for *THE SOUP CLEANSE: A Revolutionary Detox of Nourishing Soups and Healing Broths* from the Founders of Soupure (Hachette 2015), and she was featured in the award-winning documentary *Rooted In Peace* (2013).

NOTES/BIBLIOGRAPHY

INTRODUCTION: YOU GOTTA CHANGE

Understanding Acute and Chronic Inflammation. Harvard Health Publishing, Apr. 2020.

Wiss, N.A., & Rada, P. (2018). *Sugar Addiction: From Evolution to Revolution.* Front Psychiatry.

Blum, K, Thanos, K.P., & Gold, M.S. (2014). *Dopamine and glucose, obesity, and reward deficiency syndrome.* Front Psychol. 5:919.

Biological Psychology, 69(1), 5-21. Epub, 2004, Dec. 29.

Hirth, J. M., Rahman, M., & Berenson. (2002). *The association of posttraumatic stress disorder with fast food and soda consumption and unhealthy weight loss behaviors among young women.* Journal of Women's Health 20, no. 8 1141–1149.

Julson, E. (2019,). *6 Surprising Health Benefits of Sweet Potatoes.* Healthline Media, 9 Jan.

Effects of Ascorbic Acid Supplementation on Serum Progesterone Levels in Patients with a Luteal Phase Defect. Fertility and Sterility, American Society for Reproductive Medicine 80, no. 2 (2003): 459-61.

Aging Changes in the Female Reproductive System. MedlinePlus, U.S. National Library of Medicine

Regidor, P-A. (2014). *Progesterone in Peri- and Postmenopause: A Review.* Geburtshilfe und Frauenheilkunde vol. 74,11 995-1002. doi:10.1055/s-0034-1383297

Important Nutrients to Know: Proteins, Carbohydrates, and Fats. National Institute on Aging, U.S. Department of Health and Human Services.

Guan, Y., & He, Q. (2015). *Plants Consumption and Liver Health.* Evidence-based complementary and alternative medicine : eCAM 824185. doi:10.1155/2015/824185

Zhou, T., Zhang, Y. J., Xu, D. P., Wang, F., Zhou, Y., Zheng, J., Li, Y., Zhang, J. J., & Li, H. B. (2017). *Protective Effects of Lemon Juice on Alcohol-Induced Liver Injury in Mice.* BioMed Research International, 2017, 7463571. https://doi.org/10.1155/2017/7463571

Shimizu, C., Wakita, Y., Inoue, T., Hiramitsu, M., Okada, M., Mitani, Y., Segawa, S., Tsuchiya, Y., & Nabeshima, T. (2019). (*Effects of lifelong intake of lemon polyphenols on aging and intestinal microbiome in the senescence-accelerated mouse prone* 1SAMP1). Scientific reports, 9(1), 3671. https://doi.org/10.1038/s41598-019-40253-x

Nehlig, A. (2013) *The neuroprotective effects of cocoa flavanol and its influence on cognitive performance.* British Journal of Clinical Pharmacology vol. 75,3 716-27. doi:10.1111/j.1365-2125.2012.04378.x

Katz, D. L., Doughty, K., & Ali, A. (2011). *Cocoa and chocolate in human health and disease.* Antioxidants & redox signaling, 15(10), 2779–2811. https://doi.org/10.1089/ars.2010.3697

Scholey, A., & Owen, L. (2013) *Effects of chocolate on cognitive function and mood: a systematic review.* Nutrition reviews vol. 71,10 665-81. doi:10.1111/nure.12065

Chacko, S. M., Thambi, P. T., Kuttan, R., & Nishigaki, I. (2010). *Beneficial effects of green tea: a literature review.*, 5, 13. https://doi.org/10.1186/1749-8546-5-13 Chinese medicine

Pae, M., & Wu, D. (2013): *Immunomodulating effects of epigallocatechin-3-gallate from green tea: mechanisms and applications.* Food & Function vol. 4,9 1287-303. doi:10.1039/c3fo60076a

Suzuki, Y., Miyoshi, N., & Isemura, M. (2012). *Health-promoting effects of green tea.* Proceedings of the Japan Academy. Series B, Physical and Biological Sciences, 88(3), 88–101. https://doi.org/10.2183/pjab.88.88

Jain-Ping, D., Jun, C., Yu-Fei, B., Bang-Xing, H., Shang-Bin, G., & Li-Li, J. (2010). *Effects of pearl powder extract and its fractions on fibroblast function relevant to wound repair.* Pharmaceutical Biology vol. 48,2 (2010): 122-7. doi:10.3109/13880200903046211

CHAPTER 1: THE RADIANT WOMAN

Niaz, K., Zaplatic, E., and Spoor, J. (2018). *Extensive use of monosodium glutamate: A threat to public health?* EXCLI journal, *17*, 273–278. https://doi.org/10.17179/excli2018-1092

Samieri, C., Sun, Q., Townsend, M. K., Chiuve, S. E., Okereke, O. I., Willett, W. C., Stampfer, M., & Grodstein, F. (2013). *The association between dietary patterns at midlife and health in aging: an observational study.* Annals of Internal Medicine, *159*(9), 584–591. https://doi.org/10.7326/0003-4819-159-9-201311050-00004

Atallah, N., Adjibade, M., Lelong, H., Hercberg, S., Galan, P., Assmann, K. E., & Kesse-Guyot, E. (2018). *How Healthy Lifestyle Factors at Midlife Relate to Healthy Aging.* Nutrients, 10(7), 854. https://doi.org/10.3390/nu10070854

Chedraui., P, & Pérez-López, F. R. (2013) *Nutrition and health during mid-life: searching for solutions and meeting challenges for the aging population.* Climacteric : The Journal of the International Menopause Society vol. 16 Suppl 1 85-95. doi:10. 3109/13697137.2013.802884

Yau, Y-H. C., & Potenza, M. N. *Stress and Eating Behaviors.* Minerva Endocrinologica vol. 38, 3 (2013): 255-67.

Kalra, S., Jena, B. N., & Yeravdekar, R. (2018). *Emotional and Psychological Needs of People with Diabetes,* Indian Journal of Endocrinology and Metabolism, *22*(5), 696–704. https://doi.org/10.4103/ijem.IJEM_579_17

Tryon, M. S., Stanhope, K. L., Epel, E. S., Mason, A. E., Brown, R., Medici, V., Havel, P. J., & Laugero, K. D. (2015). *Excessive Sugar Consumption May Be a Difficult Habit to Break: A View From the Brain and Body.* The Journal of Clinical Endocrinology and Metabolism, *100*(6), 2239–2247. https://doi.org/10.1210/jc.2014-4353

Wahl, D. R., Villinger, K., König, L. M., Ziesemer, K., Schupp, H. T., & Renner, B. (2017). *Healthy food choices are happy food choices: Evidence from a real life sample using smartphone based assessments.* Scientific Reports, *7*(1), 17069. https://doi. org/10.1038/s41598-017-17262-9

Sathyanarayana Rao, T. S., Asha, M. R., Jagannatha Rao, K. S., & Vasudevaraju, P. (2009). *The biochemistry of belief.* Indian Journal of Psychiatry, *51*(4), 239–241. https://doi.org/10.4103/0019-5545.58285

Zaccaro, A., Piarulli, A., Laurino, M., Garbella, E., Menicucci, D., Neri, B., & Gemignani, A. (2018). *How Breath-Control Can Change Your Life: A Systematic Review on Psycho-Physiological Correlates of Slow Breathing.* Frontiers in Human Neuroscience, *12*, 353. https://doi.org/10.3389/fnhum.2018.00353

Baliga, M. S., & Dsouza, J. J. (2011). *Amla (Emblica officinalis Gaertn), a wonder berry in the treatment and prevention of cancer.* European Journal of Cancer Prevention : The Official Journal of the European Cancer Prevention Organisation (ECP) vol. 20,3 225-39. doi:10.1097/CEJ.0b013e32834473f4

Lim, D. W., Kim, J. G., & Kim, Y. T. (2016). *Analgesic Effect of Indian Gooseberry (Emblica officinalis Fruit) Extracts on Postoperative and Neuropathic Pain in Rats.* Nutrients, *8*(12), 760. https://doi.org/10.3390/nu8120760

Tarwadi, K., & Agte, V. (2007) *Antioxidant and micronutrient potential of common fruits available in the Indian subcontinent.* International Journal of Food Sciences and Nutrition vol. 58,5 341-9. doi:10.1080/09637480701243905

Akhtar MS, Ramzan A, Ali A, Ahmad M. *Effect of Amla fruit (Emblica officinalis Gaertn.) on blood glucose and lipid profile of normal subjects and type 2 diabetic patients.* Int J Food Sci Nutr. 2011;62(6):609-616. doi:10.3109/09637486.2011.560565

D'souza JJ, D'souza PP, Fazal F, Kumar A, Bhat HP, Baliga MS. *Anti-diabetic effects of the Indian indigenous fruit Emblica officinalis Gaertn: active constituents and modes of action.* Food Funct. 2014;5(4):635-644. doi:10.1039/c3fo60366k

Rao TP, Okamoto T, Akita N, Hayashi T, Kato-Yasuda N, Suzuki K. *Amla (Emblica officinalis Gaertn.) extract inhibits lipopolysaccharide-induced procoagulant and pro-inflammatory factors in cultured vascular endothelial cells.* Br J Nutr. 2013;110(12):2201-2206. doi:10.1017/S0007114513001669

Singh, M. K., Yadav, S. S., Yadav, R. S., Singh, U. S., Shukla, Y., Pant, K. K., & Khattri, S. (2014). *Efficacy of crude extract of Emblica officinalis (amla) in arsenic-induced oxidative damage and apoptosis in splenocytes of mice.* Toxicology International, *21*(1), 8–17. https://doi.org/10.4103/0971-6580.128784

Krishnaveni, M., & Mirunalini, S. (2010) *Therapeutic potential of Phyllanthus emblica (amla): the ayurvedic wonder.* Journal of Basic and Clinical Physiology and Pharmacology, vol. 21,1 93-105. doi:10.1515/jbcpp.2010.21.1.93

Wang, Y., Liu, Z., Han, Y., Xu, J., Huang, W., & Li, Z. (2018). *Medium Chain Triglycerides enhances exercise endurance through the increased mitochondrial biogenesis and metabolism.* PLOS ONE, *13*(2), e0191182. https://doi.org/10.1371/journal.pone.0191182

St-Onge, M. P., Mayrsohn, B., O'Keeffe, M., Kissileff, H. R., Choudhury, A. R., & Laferrère, B. (2014). *Impact of medium and long chain triglycerides consumption on appetite and food intake in overweight men.* European Journal of Clinical Nutrition, *68*(10), 1134–1140. https://doi.org/10.1038/ejcn.2014.145

CHAPTER 2: THE 3 C'S

Schneiderman, N., Ironson, G., & Siegel, S. D. (2005). *Stress and health: psychological, behavioral, and biological determinants.* Annual Review of Clinical Psychology, 1, 607–628. https://doi.org/10.1146/annurev.clinpsy.1.102803.144141

Yaribeygi, H., Panahi, Y., Sahraei, H., Johnston, T. P., & Sahebkar, A. (2017).

The Impact of Stress on Body Function: A Review. EXCLI Journal, 16, 1057–1072. https://doi.org/10.17179/excli2017-480

Hannibal, K. E., & Bishop, M. D. (2014). *Chronic Stress, Cortisol Dysfunction, and Pain: A Psychoneuroendocrine Rationale for Stress Management in Pain Rehabilitation.* Physical Therapy vol. 94,12 1816-25. doi:10.2522/ptj.20130597

Lenze, E. J., Mantella, R. C., Shi, P., Goate, A. M., Nowotny, P., Butters, M. A., Andreescu, C., Thompson, P. A., & Rollman, B. L. (2011). *Elevated cortisol in older adults with generalized anxiety disorder is reduced by treatment: a placebo-controlled evaluation of escitalopram.* The American journal of Geriatric Psychiatry: Official Journal of the American Association for Geriatric Psychiatry, 19(5), 482–490. https://doi.org/10.1097/JGP.0b013e3181ec806c

Yaribeygi, H., Panahi, Y., Sahraei, H., Johnston, T. P., & Sahebkar, A. (2017). *The Impact of Stress on Body Function: A Review.* EXCLI Journal, 16, 1057–1072. https://doi.org/10.17179/excli2017-480

Mariotti, A. (2015). *The Effects of Chronic Stress on Health: New Insights into the Molecular Mechanisms of Brain-Body Communication.* Future Science OA vol. 1,3 FSO23. 1 Nov. doi:10.4155/fso.15.21

Lovallo, W. R. (2006). *Cortisol Secretion Patterns in Addiction and Addiction Risk.* International Journal of Psychophysiology : Official Journal of the International Organization of Psychophysiology vol. 59,3 195-202. doi:10.1016/j. ijpsycho.2005.10.007

CHAPTER 3: THE AGING METABOLISM

Liochev, Stefan I.; Salmon, Adam (2015). *What is the Most Significant Cause of Aging?* US National Library of Medicine, National Institutes of Health, Antioxidants (Basel). Doi: 10.3390/antiox4040793, https://www.ncbi.nlm.nih.gov/pmc/articles/PMC4712935/

Fulap, Tamas; Larbi, Anis; Khalil, Abdelouahed; Cohen, Alan A.; Witkowski, Jacek M. (2019) *Are We Ill Because We Age?* frontiers in Psychology doi: 10.3389/fphys.2019.01508 https://www.ncbi.nlm.nih.gov/pmc/articles/PMC6951428/

Sánchez López de Nava, Raja, Avais (2019) *Physiology, Metabolism,* StatPearls (Internet). https://www.ncbi.nlm.nih.gov/books/NBK546690/

Guo, Chunyan. (2013). *Oxidative stress, mitochondrial damage and neurodegenerative diseases.* Neural regeneration research, *8*(21), 2003–2014. https://doi.org/10.3969/j.issn.1673-5374.2013.21.009

Lobo, V., Patil, A., Phatak, A., & Chandra, N. (2010). *Free Radicals, Antioxidants and Functional Foods: Impact on Human Health.* Pharmacognosy Reviews, *4*(8), 118–126. https://doi.org/10.4103/0973-7847.70902

Pizzomo, Joseph. (2014). *Glutathione!, Integrative Medicine, A Clinician's Journal, US National Library of Medicine,* National Institutes of Health, PMCID: PMC4684116 https://www.ncbi.nlm.nih.gov/pmc/articles/PMC4684116/

Beck, Melinda A.; Brown, David A.; Green, William D.; Shaikh, Saame Raza, Sullivan, Madison E. (2018) *Mechanisms by Which Dietary Fatty Acids Regulate Mitochondrial Structure-Function in Health and Disease,* Advances in Nutrition, US National Library of Medicine, National Institutes of Health. doi: 10.1093/advances/nmy007, PMCID: PMC5952932

PMID: 29767698 https://www.ncbi.nlm.nih.gov/pmc/articles/PMC5952932/

Bai, Li; Bao, Hongkun; Dong, Chunjie; Du, Jing; Henter, Ioline; Rudorfer, Matthew; Vitello, Benedetto; Xiao, Chunjie, Zhang, Grace Y.; *The Role of Nutrients in Protecting Mitochondrial Function and Neurotransmitter Signaling: Implications for the Treatment of Depression, PTSD, and Suicidal Behaviors,* US National Library of Medicine, National Institutes of Health. doi: 10.1080/10408398.2013.876960, PMCID: PMC4417658, NIHMSID: NIHMS653311. https://www.ncbi.nlm.nih.gov/pmc/articles/PMC4417658/

Type 2 Diabetes and Sleep Problems in Midlife Women. ScienceDaily, The North American Menopause Society (NAMS) , 14 Aug. 2019. (No Author)

Kalyani, R. R., & Egan, J. M. (2013). *Diabetes and altered glucose metabolism with aging. Endocrinology and metabolism clinics of North America*, 42(2), 333–347.

Hantzidiamantis P. J., & Lappin, S.L. (2019) *Physiology, Glucose*. [Updated Aug 13]. In: StatPearls [Internet]. Treasure Island (FL): StatPearls Publishing; 2020 Jan-.

Wilcox G. (2005). *Insulin and Insulin Resistance.* The Clinical Biochemist. American Physiological Society, Reviews, 26(2), 19–39. https://www.ncbi.nlm.nih.gov/pmc/articles/PMC6170977/

Petersen, M. C., & Shulman, G. I. (2018). *Mechanisms of Insulin Action and Insulin Resistance.* Physiological Reviews, 98(4), 2133–2223. https://doi.org/10.1152/physrev.00063.2017

Ojha, A., Ojha, U., Mohammed, R., Chandrashekar, A., & Ojha, H. (2019). *Current perspective on the role of insulin and glucagon in the pathogenesis and treatment of type 2 diabetes mellitus.* Clinical Pharmacology: Advances and Applications, 11, 57–65. https://www.ncbi.nlm.nih.gov/pmc/articles/PMC6515536/

Freeman A. M., Pennings N.(2020) *Insulin Resistance*. [Updated 2020 Jul 10]. In: StatPearls [Internet]. Treasure Island (FL): StatPearls Publishing;Jan

Jura, M., & Kozak, L. P. (2016). *Obesity and related consequences to ageing.* Age (Dordrecht, Netherlands), US National Library of Medicine, National Institutes of Health., 38(1), 23. https://doi.org/10.1007/s11357-016-9884-3

Swarup S, Goyal A, Grigorova Y, & Zeltser R. (2020) *Metabolic Syndrome.* [Updated 2020 May 20]. In: StatPearls [Internet]. Treasure Island (FL): StatPearls Publishing.

Navarro-Pardo, E., Holland, C. A., & Cano, A. (2018). *Sex Hormones and Healthy Psychological Aging in Women.* Frontiers in Aging Neuroscience, 9, 439. https://www.ncbi.nlm.nih.gov/pmc/articles/PMC5767260/

Horstman, A. M., Dillon, E. L., Urban, R. J., & Sheffield-Moore, M. (2012). *The Role of Androgens and Estrogens on Healthy Aging and Longevity.* The Journals of Gerontology. Series A, Biological Sciences and Medical Sciences, 67(11), 1140–1152. https://www.ncbi.nlm.nih.gov/pmc/articles/PMC3636678/

Schwarz, N. A., Rigby, B. R., La Bounty, P., Shelmadine, B., & Bowden, R. G. (2011). *A Review of Weight Control Strategies and Their Effects on the Regulation of Hormonal Balance.* Journal of Nutrition and Metabolism, 2011, 237932. https://doi.org/10.1155/2011/237932

Liu, G., Liang, L., Bray, G. A., Qi, L., Hu, F. B., Rood, J., Sacks, F. M., & Sun, Q. (2017). *Thyroid Hormones and Changes in Body Weight and Metabolic Parameters in Response to Weight Loss Diets: the POUNDS LOST Trial.* International Journal of Obesity (2005), 41(6), 878–886. https://doi.org/10.1038/ijo.2017.28

Janssen, I., Powell, L. H., Kazlauskaite, R., & Dugan, S. A. (2010). *Testosterone and visceral fat in midlife women: The Study of Women's Health Across the Nation (SWAN) fat patterning study.* Obesity, A Research Journal, (Silver Spring, Md.), 18(3), 604–610. https://onlinelibrary.wiley.com/doi/full/10.1038/oby.2009.251

Kelesidis, T., Kelesidis, I., Chou, S., & Mantzoros, C. S. (2010). *Narrative Review: The Role of Leptin in Human Physiology: Emerging Clinical Applications.* Annals of Internal Medicine, 152(2), 93–100. https://doi.org/10.7326/0003-4819-152-2-201001190-00008

Gruzdeva, O., Borodkina, D., Uchasova, E., Dyleva, Y., & Barbarash, O. (2019). *Leptin resistance: underlying mechanisms and diagnosis. Diabetes, metabolic syndrome and obesity : targets and therapy,* 12, 191–198. https://doi.org/10.2147/DMSO.S182406

Smith, A. J., Giunta, B., Shytle, R. D., & Blum, J. M. (2011). *Evaluation of a novel supplement to reduce blood glucose through the use of a modified oral glucose tolerance test.* American Journal of Translational Research, 3(2), 219–225. https://www.ncbi.nlm.nih.gov/pmc/articles/PMC5078644/

Pintaudi, B., Di Vieste, G., & Bonomo, M. (2016). *The Effectiveness of Myo-Inositol and D-Chiro Inositol Treatment in Type 2 Diabetes.* International Journal of Endocrinology, 2016, 9132052. https://doi.org/10.1155/2016/9132052

Cao, C., & Su, M. (2019). *Effects of berberine on glucose-lipid metabolism, inflammatory factors and insulin resistance in patients with metabolic syndrome.* Experimental and therapeutic medicine, 17(4), 3009–3014. https://doi.org/10.3892/etm.2019.7295

Lepretti, M., Martucciello, S., Burgos Aceves, M. A., Putti, R., & Lionetti, L. (2018*). Omega-3 Fatty Acids and Insulin Resistance: Focus on the Regulation of Mitochondria and Endoplasmic Reticulum Stress.* Nutrients, 10(3), 350. https://doi.org/10.3390/nu10030350

Wend, K., Wend, P., & Krum, S. A. (2012). *Tissue-Specific Effects of Loss of Estrogen during Menopause and Aging. Frontiers in endocrinology*, 3, 19. https://doi.org/10.3389/fendo.2012.00019

Peacock K, Ketvertis K. M.(2020) *Menopause.* [Updated 2020 Aug 16]. In: StatPearls [Internet]. Treasure Island (FL): StatPearls Publishing;Jan-.

Fait T. (2019). *Menopause hormone therapy: latest developments and clinical practice.* Drugs in Context, 8, 212551. https://doi.org/10.7573/dic.212551

Iorga, A., Cunningham, C. M., Moazeni, S., Ruffenach, G., Umar, S., & Eghbali, M. (2017*). The protective role of estrogen and estrogen receptors in cardiovascular disease and the controversial use of estrogen therapy.* Biology of Sex Differences, 8(1), 33. https://doi.org/10.1186/s13293-017-0152-8

Paterni, I., Granchi, C., & Minutolo, F. (2017). *Risks and benefits related to alimentary exposure to xenoestrogens.* Critical Reviews in Food Science and Nutrition, 57(16), 3384–3404. https://doi.org/10.1080/10408398.2015.1126547

Fucic, A., Gamulin, M., Ferencic, Z., Katic, J., Krayer von Krauss, M., Bartonova, A., & Merlo, D. F. (2012). *Environmental exposure to xenoestrogens and oestrogen related cancers: reproductive system, breast, lung, kidney, pancreas, and brain.* Environmental Health: A Global Access Science Source, 11 Suppl 1(Suppl 1), S8. https://doi.org/10.1186/1476-069X-11-S1-S8

Samavat, H., & Kurzer, M. S. (2015). *Estrogen metabolism and breast cancer.* Cancer Letters, 356(2 Pt A), 231–243. https://doi.org/10.1016/j.canlet.2014.04.018

Rajoria, S., R. Suriano, P.S. Parmar, Y. L. Wilson, U. Megwalu, a. Moscatello, H. L. Bradlow, D. W. Sepkovic, J. Geliebte, S. P. Schantz, & R. K. Tiware (2011). *3,3'-diindolylmethane modulates estrogen metabolism in patients with thyroid proliferative disease: a pilot study.* Thyroid 21(3); 299-304.

Smith, R. L., Gallicchio, L., & Flaws, J. A. (2017). *Factors Affecting Sexual Function in Midlife Women: Results from the Midlife Women's Health Study.* Journal of Women's Health (2002), 26(9), 923–932. https://doi.org/10.1089/jwh.2016.6135

Sarkar, M., Wellons, M., Cedars, M. I., VanWagner, L., Gunderson, E. P., Ajmera, V., Torchen, L., Siscovick, D., Carr, J. J., Terry, J. G., Rinella, M., Lewis, C. E., & Terrault, N. (2017). *Testosterone Levels in Pre-Menopausal Women are Associated With Nonalcoholic Fatty Liver Disease in Midlife.* The American journal of Gastroenterology, 112(5), 755–762. https://doi.org/10.1038/ajg.2017.44

Grube, BJ., Eng, E. T., Kao, Y. C., Kwon, A, & Chen, S. (2001) . *White Button Mushroom,* J Nutr. December vol 131 no. 12;3288-93.

Kostoglou-Athanassiou I. (2013). Therapeutic applications of melatonin. Therapeutic advances in endocrinology and metabolism, 4(1), 13–24. https://doi.org/10.1177/2042018813476084

Peuhkuri, K., Sihvola, N., & Korpela, R. (2012). *Dietary factors and fluctuating levels of melatonin.* Food & nutrition research, 56, 10.3402/fnr.v56i0.17252. https://doi.org/10.3402/fnr.v56i0.17252

Samaras, N., Samaras, D., Frangos, E., Forster, A., & Philippe, J. (2013). *A Review of Age-related Dehydroepiandrosterone Decline and Its Association with Well-known Geriatric Syndromes: Is Treatment Beneficial?* Rejuvenation Research, 16(4), 285–294. https://doi.org/10.1089/rej.2013.1425

Lavretsky, H., & Newhouse, P. A. (2012). *Stress, Inflammation, and Aging.* The American Journal of Geriatric Psychiatry: Official Journal of the American Association for Geriatric Psychiatry, 20(9), 729–733. https://doi.org/10.1097/JGP.0b013e31826573cf

Dedovic, K., & Ngiam, J. (2015). *The cortisol awakening response and major depression: examining the evidence.* Neuropsychiatric disease and treatment vol. 11 1181-9. 14 May. doi:10.2147/NDT.S62289

Trefts, E., Gannon, M., & Wasserman, D. H. (2017). The liver. Current Biology : CB, 27(21), R1147–R1151. https://doi.org/10.1016/j.cub.2017.09.019

Chung, H. Y., Kim, D. H., Lee, E. K., Chung, K. W., Chung, S., Lee, B., Seo, A. Y., Chung, J. H., Jung, Y. S., Im, E., Lee, J., Kim, N. D., Choi, Y. J., Im, D. S., & Yu, B. P. (2019). *Redefining Chronic Inflammation in Aging and Age-Related Diseases: Proposal of the Senoinflammation Concept.* Aging and Disease, 10(2), 367–382. https://doi.org/10.14336/AD.2018.0324

Sanada, F., Taniyama, Y., Muratsu, J., Otsu, R., Shimizu, H., Rakugi, H., & Morishita, R. (2018). *Source of Chronic Inflammation in Aging.* Frontiers in Cardiovascular Medicine, 5, 12. https://doi.org/10.3389/fcvm.2018.00012

Rea, I. M., Gibson, D. S., McGilligan, V., McNerlan, S. E., Alexander, H. D., & Ross, O. A. (2018). *Age and Age-Related Diseases: Role of Inflammation Triggers and Cytokines.* Frontiers in Immunology, 9, 586. https://doi.org/10.3389/fimmu.2018.00586

Aubert G, Lansdorp P. M. *Telomeres and Aging.* Physiol Rev. 2008;88(2):557-579. doi:10.1152/physrev.00026.2007

Belkaid, Y., & Hand, T. W. (2014). *Role of the Microbiota in Immunity and Inflammation.* Cell, 157(1), 121–141. https://doi.org/10.1016/j.cell.2014.03.011

O'Callaghan, A., & Sinderen, D. V. (2016). *Bifidobacteria and Their Role as Members of the Human Gut Microbiota.* Frontiers in microbiology vol. 7 925. 15 Jun., doi:10.3389/fmicb.2016.00925

Lloyd-Price, J., Abu-Ali, G., & Huttenhower, C. (2016). *The Healthy Human Microbiome.* Genome Medicine, 8(1), 51. https://doi.org/10.1186/s13073-016-0307-y

Bull, M. J., & Plummer, N. T. (2014). *Part 1: The Human Gut Microbiome in Health and Disease.* Integrative medicine (Encinitas, Calif.), 13(6), 17–22.

Jandhyala, S. M., Talukdar, R., Subramanyam, C., Vuyyuru, H., Sasikala, M., & Nageshwar Reddy, D. (2015). *Role of the normal gut microbiota.* World journal of Gastroenterology, 21(29), 8787–8803. https://doi.org/10.3748/wjg.v21.i29.8787

Can Gut Bacteria Improve Your Health? Harvard Men's Health Watch, Harvard Health Publishing, Oct. 2016. (No author) https://www.ncbi.nlm.nih.gov/pmc/articles/PMC3983973/

Quigley E. M. (2013). *Gut bacteria in health and disease.* Gastroenterology & Hepatology, 9(9), 560–569.

Makki K, Deehan, E. C., Walter J, Bäckhed F. *The Impact of Dietary Fiber on Gut Microbiota in Host Health and Disease.* Cell Host Microbe. 2018;23(6):705-715. doi:10.1016/j.chom.2018.05.012 https://www.ncbi.nlm.nih.gov/pmc/articles/PMC7146107/

Myhrstad, M., Tunsjø, H., Charnock, C., & Telle-Hansen, V. H. (2020). *Dietary Fiber, Gut Microbiota, and Metabolic Regulation-Current Status in Human Randomized Trials.* Nutrients, 12(3), 859. https://doi.org/10.3390/nu12030859

Den Besten, G., Van Eunen, K., Groen, A. K., Venema, K., Reijngoud, D. J., & Bakker, B. M. (2013). *The role of short-chain fatty acids in the interplay between diet, gut microbiota, and host energy metabolism.* Journal of Lipid Research, 54(9), 2325–2340

Liu, H., Wang, J., He, T., Becker, S., Zhang, G., Li, D., & Ma, X. (2018). *Butyrate: A Double-Edged Sword for Health?* Advances in Nutrition (Bethesda, Md.) vol. 9,1 21-29. doi:10.1093/advances/nmx009

Kowiański, P., Lietzau, G., Czuba, E., Waśkow, M., Steliga, A., & Moryś, J. (2018). *BDNF: A Key Factor with Multipotent Impact on Brain Signaling and Synaptic Plasticity.* Cellular and Molecular Neurobiology, 38(3), 579–593. https://doi.org/10.1007/s10571-017-0510-4

Binder, D. K., & Scharfman, H. E. (2004). *Brain-derived neurotrophic factor.* Growth factors (Chur, Switzerland) vol. 22,3, 123-31. doi:10.1080/08977190410001723308

Davani-Davari, D., Negahdaripour, M., Karimzadeh, I., Seifan, M., Mohkam, M., Masoumi, S. J., Berenjian, A., & Ghasemi, Y. (2019). *Prebiotics: Definition, Types, Sources, Mechanisms, and Clinical Applications.* Foods (Basel, Switzerland), 8(3), 92. https://doi.org/10.3390/foods8030092

Holscher H. D. (2017). *Dietary fiber and prebiotics and the gastrointestinal microbiota. Gut microbes,* 8(2), 172–184. https://doi.org/10.1080/19490976.2017.1290756

Birt, D. F., Boylston, T., Hendrich, S., Jane, J. L., Hollis, J., Li, L., McClelland, J., Moore, S., Phillips, G. J., Rowling, M., Schalinske, K., Scott, M. P., & Whitley, E. M. (2013). *Resistant Starch: Promise for Improving Human Health.* Advances in Nutrition (Bethesda, Md.), 4(6), 587–601. https://doi.org/10.3945/an.113.004325

Maier, T. V., Lucio, M., Lee, L. H., VerBerkmoes, N. C., Brislawn, C. J., Bernhardt, J., Lamendella, R., McDermott, J. E., Bergeron, N., Heinzmann, S. S., Morton, J. T., González, A., Ackermann, G., Knight, R., Riedel, K., Krauss, R. M., Schmitt-Kopplin, P., & Jansson, J. K. (2017). *Impact of Dietary Resistant Starch on the Human Gut Microbiome, Metaproteome, and Metabolome.* mBio, 8(5), e01343-17. https://doi.org/10.1128/mBio.01343-17

Bindels, L. B., Segura Munoz, R. R., Gomes-Neto, J. C., Mutemberezi, V., Martínez, I., Salazar, N., Cody, E. A., Quintero-Villegas, M. I., Kittana, H., de Los Reyes-Gavilán, C. G., Schmaltz, R. J., Muccioli, G. G., Walter, J., & Ramer-Tait, A. E. (2017). *Resistant starch can improve insulin sensitivity independently of the gut microbiota.* Microbiome, 5(1), 12. https://doi.org/10.1186/s40168-017-0230-5

Trachsel, J., Briggs, C., Gabler, N. K., Allen, H. K., & Loving, C. L. (2019). *Dietary Resistant Potato Starch Alters Intestinal Microbial Communities and Their Metabolites, and Markers of Immune Regulation and Barrier Function in Swine.* Frontiers in immunology, 10, 1381. https://doi.org/10.3389/fimmu.2019.01381

Hemarajata, P., & Versalovic, J. (2013). *Effects of probiotics on gut microbiota: mechanisms of intestinal immunomodulation and neuromodulation.* Therapeutic Advances in Gastroenterology, 6(1), 39–51. https://doi.org/10.1177/1756283X12459294

Wieërs, G., Belkhir, L., Enaud, R., Leclercq, S., Philippart de Foy, J. M., Dequenne, I., de Timary, P., & Cani, P. D. (2020). *How Probiotics Affect the Microbiota.* frontiers in Cellular and Infection Microbiology, 9, 454. https://doi.org/10.3389/fcimb.2019.00454

Rezac, S., Kok, C. R., Heermann, M., & Hutkins, R. (2018). *Fermented Foods as a Dietary Source of Live Organisms.* Frontiers in Microbiology, 9, 1785. https://doi.org/10.3389/fmicb.2018.01785

How to Get More Probiotics. Harvard Health Publishing: Harvard Medical School. (No author), https://www.ncbi.nlm.nih.gov/pmc/articles/PMC5483960/

Wen, L., & Duffy, A. (2017*). Factors Influencing the Gut Microbiota, Inflammation, and Type 2 Diabetes.* The Journal of Nutrition, 147(7), 1468S–1475S. https://doi.org/10.3945/jn.116.240754

Hasan, N., & Yang, H. (2019). *Factors affecting the composition of the gut microbiota, and its modulation.* PeerJ, 7, e7502. https://doi.org/10.7717/peerj.7502

Appleton J. (2018). *The Gut-Brain Axis: Influence of Microbiota on Mood and Mental Health. Integrative Medicine* (Encinitas, Calif.), 17(4), 28–32. https://www.ncbi.nlm.nih.gov/pmc/articles/PMC6306769/

Skonieczna-Żydecka, K., Marlicz, W., Misera, A., Koulaouzidis, A., & Łoniewski, I. (2018). *Microbiome-The Missing Link in the Gut-Brain Axis: Focus on Its Role in Gastrointestinal and Mental Health.* Journal of Clinical Medicine, 7(12), 521. https://doi.org/10.3390/jcm7120521

Fasano A. (2012). *Zonulin, regulation of tight junctions, and autoimmune diseases.* Annals of the New York Academy of Sciences, 1258(1), 25–33. https://doi.org/10.1111/j.1749-6632.2012.06538.x

Guo, S., & Dipietro, L. A. (2010). *Factors Affecting Wound Healing.* Journal of Dental Research, 89(3), 219–229. https://doi.org/10.1177/0022034509359125

Stockman, M. C., Thomas, D., Burke, J., & Apovian, C. M. (2018). *Intermittent Fasting: Is the Wait Worth the Weight?* Current Obesity Reports, 7(2), 172–185. https://doi.org/10.1007/s13679-018-0308-9

Jacomin, A. C., Gul, L., Sudhakar, P., Korcsmaros, T., & Nezis, I. P. (2018). *What We Learned from Big Data for Autophagy Research.* Frontiers in Cell and Developmental Biology, 6, 92. https://doi.org/10.3389/fcell.2018.00092

Condello, M., Pellegrini, E., Caraglia, M., & Meschini, S. (2019). *Targeting Autophagy to Overcome Human Diseases.* International Journal of Molecular Sciences, 20(3), 725. https://doi.org/10.3390/ijms20030725

Adult Obesity Facts. Centers for Disease Control and Prevention, 29 June 2020. (No author). https://www.cdc.gov/obesity/adult/defining.html

Defining Adult Overweight and Obesity. Centers for Disease Control and Prevention, 30 June 2020 (No author). https://pubmed.ncbi.nlm.nih.gov/17964227/

Rattan S. I. *Hormesis in Aging.* Ageing Res Rev. 2008;7(1):63-78. doi:10.1016/j.arr.2007.03.002

CHAPTER 4: BLOOD DOESN'T LIE

Asif M. (2014). *The prevention and control the type-2 diabetes by changing lifestyle and dietary pattern.* Journal of education and health promotion, 3, 1. https://doi.org/10.4103/2277-9531.127541

Should You Seek Advanced Cholesterol Testing? Harvard Medical School, Harvard Health Publishing, May 2014 (No author)

Kulkarni K. R. (2006). *Cholesterol Profile Measurement by Vertical Auto Profile Method.* Clinics in Laboratory Medicine, *26*(4), 787–802. https://doi.org/10.1016/j.cll.2006.07.004

Feingold K. R, Grunfeld, C. (2000-.) *Utility of Advanced Lipoprotein Testing in Clinical Practice.* [Updated 2019 Nov 5]. In: Feingold KR, Anawalt B, Boyce A, editors. Endotext[Internet]. South Dartmouth (MA): MDText.com, Inc.;

Chandra, A., & Rohatgi, A. (2014). *The Role of Advanced Lipid Testing in the Prediction of Cardiovascular Disease.* Current atherosclerosis reports, *16*(3), 394. https://doi.org/10.1007/s11883-013-0394-9

Ivanova, E. A., Myasoedova, V. A., Melnichenko, A. A., Grechko, A. V., & Orekhov, A. N. (2017). *Small Dense Low-Density Lipoprotein as Biomarker for Atherosclerotic Diseases.* Oxidative medicine and cellular longevity, *2017*, 1273042. https://doi.org/10.1155/2017/1273042

Pizzini, A., Lunger, L., Demetz, E., Hilbe, R., Weiss, G., Ebenbichler, C., & Tancevski, I. (2017). *The Role of Omega-3 Fatty Acids in Reverse Cholesterol Transport: A Review.* Nutrients, *9*(10), 1099. https://doi.org/10.3390/nu9101099

Yanai, H., Masui, Y., Katsuyama, H., Adachi, H., Kawaguchi, A., Hakoshima, M., Waragai, Y., Harigae, T., & Sako, A. (2018). *An Improvement of Cardiovascular Risk Factors by Omega-3 Polyunsaturated Fatty Acids.* Journal of Clinical Medicine Research, *10*(4), 281–289. https://doi.org/10.14740/jocmr3362w

Rosenthal R. L. (2000). *Effectiveness of Altering Serum Cholesterol Levels without Drugs.* Proceedings (Baylor University. Medical Center*)*, *13*(4), 351–355. https://doi.org/10.1080/08998280.2000.11927704

Mathew, T. K, Tadi, P. (2020). *Blood Glucose Monitoring.* [Updated 2020 Mar 28]. In: StatPearls [Internet]. Treasure Island (FL): StatPearls Publishing; Jan-.

Owora A. H. (2018). *Commentary: Diagnostic Validity and Clinical Utility of HbA1c Tests for Type 2 Diabetes Mellitus.* Current Diabetes Reviews, *14*(2), 196–199. https://doi.org/10.2174/1573399812666161129154559

Eyth, E., Naik, R., (2020). *Hemoglobin A1C.* [Updated 2020 Jan 31]. In: StatPearls [Internet]. Treasure Island (FL): StatPearlsPublishing; Jan-.

Sami, W., Ansari, T., Butt, N. S., & Hamid, M. (2017). *Effect of Diet on Type 2 Diabetes Mellitus: A review.* International Journal of Health Sciences, *11*(2), 65–71.

InformedHealth.org [Internet]. Cologne, Germany: Institute for Quality and Efficiency in Health Care (IQWiG); 2006-. *How does the thyroid gland work?* 2010 Nov 17 [Updated 2018 Apr 19].

Mullur, R., Liu, Y. Y., & Brent, G. A. (2014). *Thyroid Hormone Regulation of Metabolism.* Physiological Reviews, *94*(2), 355–382. https://doi.org/10.1152/physrev.00030.2013

Armstrong, M., Asuka, E., Fingeret , A. (2020). *Physiology, Thyroid Function.* [Updated 2020 May 21]. In: StatPearls [Internet]. Treasure Island (FL): StatPearls Publishing; Jan-.

Gomes-Lima, C., Wartofsky, L., & Burman, K. (2019). *Can Reverse T3 Assay Be Employed to Guide T4 vs. T4/T3 Therapy in Hypothyroidism?* Frontiers in Endocrinology, *10*, 856. https://doi.org/10.3389/fendo.2019.00856

Shimada T. (1984). *Nihon Naibunpi Gakkai zasshi, 60*(3), 195–206. https://doi.org/10.1507/endocrine1927.60.3_195

Senese, R., Cioffi, F., de Lange, P., Goglia, F., & Lanni, A. (2014). *Thyroid: Biological Actions of 'Nonclassical' Thyroid Hormones.* The Journal of Endocrinology, *221*(2), R1–R12. https://doi.org/10.1530/JOE-13-0573

Peeters, R. P., Wouters, P. J., van Toor, H., Kaptein, E., Visser, T. J., & Van den Berghe, G. (2005). *Serum 3,3',5'-triiodothyronine (rT3) and 3,5,3'-triiodothyronine/ rT3 are Prognostic Markers in Critically Ill Patients and are Associated with Postmortem Tissue Deiodinase Activities.* The Journal of Clinical Endocrinology and Metabolism, *90*(8), 4559–4565. https://doi.org/10.1210/jc.2005-0535

Mariotti, S.(2005). *Editorial: Thyroid Function and Aging: Do Serum 3,5,3-Triiodothyronine and Thyroid-Stimulating Hormone Concentrations Give the*

Janus Response?, The Journal of Clinical Endocrinology & Metabolism, Volume 90, Issue 12, 1 December, Pages 6735–6737,https://doi.org/10.1210/jc.2005-2214

Andrade, G., Gorgulho, B., Lotufo, P. A., Bensenor, I. M., & Marchioni, D. M. (2018). *Dietary Selenium Intake and Subclinical Hypothyroidism: A Cross-Sectional Analysis of the ELSA-Brasil Study.* Nutrients, *10*(6), 693. https://doi.org/10.3390/nu10060693

Babiker, A., Alawi, A., Al Atawi, M., & Al Alwan, I. (2020). *The Role of Micronutrients in Thyroid Dysfunction.* Sudanese Journal of Paediatrics, *20*(1), 13–19. https://doi.org/10.24911/SJP.106-1587138942

Peacock, K., Ketvertis, K. M. (2020). [Updated 2020 Apr 27]. In: StatPearls [Internet]. Treasure Island (FL): StatPearls Publishing; Jan-.

Kloss, K. (2020). *"Hormone Imbalance and Menopause. Hormone Level Testing."* Health Testing Centers, 29 Apr.

CHAPTER 5: NEXT LEVEL NUTRITION

CFR - Code of Federal Regulations Title 21. US Food and Drug Administration , US Department of Health and Human Services , 1 Apr. 2019. (No author)

Tadvi, N. (2013) *Excitotoxins: Their Role in Health and Disease.* Research Gate, July .IJMRHS. 2. 648-59. 10.5958/j.2319-5886.2.3.047

University of North Carolina at Chapel Hill. *MSG Use Linked To Obesity.* ScienceDaily. ScienceDaily, 14 August 2008. (No author)

American University. *Pilot Study in Kenya Shows Link Between Chronic Pain and Glutamate Consumption: Researchers Test Theory that Diet Change Can Alleviate Pain.* ScienceDaily. ScienceDaily, 16 February 2018. (No author)

The International Classification of Headache Disorders, 3rd Edition." Cephalalgia, International Headache Society, 2013. (No author)

Hossam, A. S., Elgohary, A. A, Metwally, F. G., Moustafa S., & Sayed, A. A. (2012). *Monosodium Glutamate-induced Damage in Rabbit Retina: Electroretinographic and Histologic Studies.*

Olney, J. W. (1969). *Brain Lesions, Obesity, and Other Disturbances in Mice Treated with Monosodium Glutamate.* American Association for the Advancement of Science, 9 May

Blaylock, R. (2020). *Excitotoxins, Neurodegeneration and Neurodevelopment*

Niaz, K., Zaplatic, E., & Spoor, J. (2018). *Extensive use of Monosodium Glutamate: A threat to Public Health?* EXCLI Journal, *17*, 273–278. https://doi.org/10.17179/excli2018-1092

Araujo, T. R., Freitas, I. N., Vettorazzi, J. F., Batista, T. M., Santos-Silva, J. C., Bonfleur, M. L., Balbo, S. L., Boschero, A. C., Carneiro, E. M., & Ribeiro, R. A. (2017). *MSG Benefits of L-alanine or L-arginine supplementation against adiposity and glucose intolerance in monosodium glutamate-induced obesity.* Eur J Nutr. Sep; 56(6):2069-2080.

He, K., Du, S., Xun, P., Sharma, S., Wang, H., Zhai, F., Popkin, B., Am, J. (2011) MSG *Consumption of monosodium glutamate in relation to incidence of overweight in Chinese adults: China Health and Nutrition Survey* (CHNS). Clin Nutr. Jun; 93(6):1328-36.

Effects of Adaptogens on the Central Nervous System and the Molecular Mechanisms Associated with their Stress - Protective Activity. Pharmaceuticals (Basel) v.3(1): 2010 Jan PMC3991026 – ADAPTOGENS

CHAPTER 6: MARLYN'S METHOD (FOR MIDLIFE!)

Barraclough, E. L., Hay-Smith, E., Boucher, S. E., Tylka, T. L., & Horwath, C. C. (2019). *Learning to eat intuitively: A qualitative exploration of the experience of mid-age women.* Health Psychology Open, 6(1), 2055102918824064. https://doi.org/10.1177/2055102918824064

Hazzard, V. M., Telke, S. E., Simone, M., Anderson, L. M., Larson, N. I., & Neumark-Sztainer, D. (2020). *Intuitive eating longitudinally predicts better psychological health and lower use of disordered eating behaviors: findings from EAT 2010-2018. Eating and weight disorders : EWD*, 10.1007/s40519-020-00852-4. Advance online publication. https://doi.org/10.1007/s40519-020-00852-4

Outland, L. (2010) *Intuitive eating: a holistic approach to weight control.* Holistic nursing practice vol. 24,1 35-43. doi:10.1097/HNP.0b013e3181c8e560

Van Dyke, N., & Drinkwater, E. J. (2014). *Relationships between intuitive eating and health indicators: literature review.* Public health nutrition vol. 17,8 1757-66. doi:10.1017/S1368980013002139

Cadena-Schlam, L., & Gemma, L-G. (2014). *Intuitive eating: an emerging approach to eating behavior.* Nutricion hospitalaria vol. 31,3 995-1002. 3 Oct. doi:10.3305/nh.2015.31.3.7980

Ruzanska, U. A., & Warschburger, P. (2019). *Intuitive eating mediates the relationship between self-regulation and BMI - Results from a cross-sectional study in a community sample.* Eating behaviors vol. 33 23-29. doi:10.1016/j.eatbeh.2019.02.004

Mayer, E. A. (2011) *Gut feelings: the emerging biology of gut-brain communication.* Nature reviews. Neuroscience vol. 12,8 453-66. 13 Jul. doi:10.1038/nrn3071

Ho, P. & Ross, D.A. (2017). *More Than a Gut Feeling: The Implications of the Gut Microbiota in Psychiatry.* Biological psychiatry vol. 81,5 e35-e37. doi:10.1016/j.biopsych.2016.12.018

Nelson, J. B. (2017). *Mindful Eating: The Art of Presence While You Eat.* Diabetes spectrum : a publication of the American Diabetes Association vol. 30,3 171-174. doi:10.2337/ds17-0015

Morillo Sarto, H., Barcelo-Soler, A., Herrera-Mercadal, P., Pantilie, B., Navarro-Gil, M., Garcia-Campayo, J., & Montero-Marin, J. (2019). *Efficacy of a mindful-eating programme to reduce emotional eating in patients suffering from overweight or obesity in primary care settings: a cluster-randomised trial protocol. BMJ open*, 9(11), e031327. https://doi.org/10.1136/bmjopen-2019-031327

Mantzios, M. & Wilson, J. C. (2015). *Mindfulness, Eating Behaviours, and Obesity: A Review and Reflection on Current Findings.* Current obesity reports vol. 4,1 141-6. doi:10.1007/s13679-014-0131-x

Janssen, L. K., Duif, I., van Loon, I., de Vries, J., Speckens, A., Cools, R., & Aarts, E. (2018). *Greater mindful eating practice is associated with better reversal learning.* Scientific reports, *8*(1), 5702. https://doi.org/10.1038/s41598-018-24001-1

Agrawal, A. K., Yadav, C. R., & Meena, M. S. (2010). *Physiological aspects of Agni.* Ayu, *31*(3), 395–398. https://doi.org/10.4103/0974-8520.77159

Steer, E. (2019). *A cross comparison between Ayurvedic etiology of Major Depressive Disorder and bidirectional effect of gut dysregulation.* Journal of Ayurveda and Integrative Medicine vol. 10,159-66. doi:10.1016/j.jaim.2017.08.002

Eswaran, H. T., Kavita, M. B., Tripaty, T. B., & Shivakumar (2015). *Formation and validation of questionnaire to assess* Jātharāgni. Ancient science of life, *34*(4), 203–209. https://doi.org/10.4103/0257-7941.159829

Food Forum; Food and Nutrition Board; Institute of Medicine. *Relationships Among the Brain, the Digestive System, and Eating Behavior: Workshop Summary.* Washington (DC): National Academies Press (US); 2015 Feb 27. 2, Interaction Between the Brain and the Digestive System.

Breton, J., Tennoune, N., Lucas, N., Francois, M., Legrand, R., Jacquemot, J., Goichon, A., Guérin, C., Peltier, J., Pestel-Caron, M., Chan, P., Vaudry, D., do Rego, J. C., Liénard, F., Pénicaud, L., Fioramonti, X., Ebenezer, I. S., Hökfelt, T., Déchelotte, P., & Fetissov, S. O. (2016). *Gut Commensal E. coli Proteins Activate Host Satiety Pathways following Nutrient-Induced Bacterial Growth.* Cell Metabolism, *23*(2), 324–334. https://doi.org/10.1016/j.cmet.2015.10.017

Barnes, S., Prasain, J., & Kim, H. (2013). *In nutrition, can we "see" what is good for us?* Advances in Nutrition *(Bethesda, Md.),* *4*(3), 327S–34S. https://doi.org/10.3945/an.112.003558

Khoo, H. E., Azlan, A., Tang, S. T., & Lim, S. M. (2017). *Anthocyanidins and anthocyanins: colored pigments as food, pharmaceutical ingredients, and the potential health benefits.* food & nutrition research, *61*(1), 1361779. https://doi.org/10.1080/16546628.2017.1361779

Liu, R. H. (2013). *Health-promoting components of fruits and vegetables in the diet.* Advances in Nutrition (Bethesda, Md.) vol. 4,3 384S-92S. 1 May. doi:10.3945/an.112.003517

Konczak, I. & Zhang, W. (2004). *Anthocyanins-More Than Nature's Colours.* Journal of Biomedicine & Biotechnology vol. 2004,5 239-240. doi:10.1155/S1110724304407013

Sarker, U. & Oba, S. (2019). *Antioxidant constituents of three selected red and green color Amaranthus leafy vegetable.* Scientific reports vol. 9,1 18233. 3 Dec. doi:10.1038/s41598-019-52033-8

Pandey, K. B., & Rizvi, S. I. (2009). *Plant polyphenols as dietary antioxidants in human health and disease*, Oxidative medicine and cellular longevity vol. 2,5 270-8. doi:10.4161/oxim.2.5.9498

Cory, H., Passarelli, S., Szeto, J., Tamez, M., & Mattei, J. (2018). *The Role of Polyphenols in Human Health and Food Systems: A Mini-Review.* frontiers in Nutrition, *5*, 87. https://doi.org/10.3389/fnut.2018.00087

Williamson, G. (2017). *The Role of Polyphenols in Modern Nutrition.* Nutrition Bulletin vol. 42,3 226-235. doi:10.1111/nbu.12278

Slavin, J. L., & Lloyd, B. (2012). *Health benefits of fruits and vegetables.* Advances in nutrition (Bethesda, Md.) vol. 3,4 506-16. 1 Jul. doi:10.3945/an.112.002154

Skerrett, P. J., and Willett, W. C. (2010): *Essentials of Healthy Eating: a Guide.* Journal of Midwifery & Women's Health vol. 55,6 492-501. doi:10.1016/j.jmwh.2010.06.019

Abuajah, C. I., Ogbonna, A. C., & Osuji, C. M. (2015). *Functional components and medicinal properties of food: a review.* Journal of Food Science and Technology, *52*(5), 2522–2529. https://doi.org/10.1007/s13197-014-1396-5

Wild Caught vs. Farm Raised Seafood. Colorado State University: College of Health and Human Sciences, Kendall Reagan Nutrition Center, 17 Apr. 2018. (No author)

Hartnell, R. *What Are the Benefits of Wild-Caught Fish over Farm Fish? Vital Choice - Wild Seafood & Organics*

Simon, D. R. & Knudsen, M. (2020). *7 Things Everyone Should Know About Farmed Fish.* Mind Body Green Food, 25 Mar.

Romagnolo, D. F., & Selmin, O. I., (2017). *Mediterranean Diet and Prevention of Chronic Diseases.* Nutrition Today vol. 52,5 208-222. doi:10.1097/NT.000000000000022

Lăcătușu, C. M., Grigorescu, E. D., Floria, M., Onofriescu, A., & Mihai, B. M. (2019). *The Mediterranean Diet: From an Environment-Driven Food Culture to an Emerging Medical Prescription.* International Journal of Environmental Research and Public Health, *16*(6), 942. https://doi.org/10.3390/ijerph16060942

Martínez-González, M. A. (2016). *Benefits of the Mediterranean diet beyond the Mediterranean Sea and beyond food patterns.* BMC Medicine vol. 14,1 157. 14 Oct. doi:10.1186/s12916-016-0714-3

Tosti, V., Bertozzi, B., & Fontana, L. (2018*).* Health Benefits of the Mediterranean Diet: Metabolic and Molecular Mechanisms. The Journals of Gerontology. Series A, Biological Sciences and Medical Sciences, *73*(3), 318–326. https://doi.org/10.1093/gerona/glx227

Franquesa, M., Pujol-Busquets, G., García-Fernández, E., Rico, L., Shamirian-Pulido, L., Aguilar-Martínez, A., Medina, F. X., Serra-Majem, L., & Bach-Faig, A. (2019). *Mediterranean Diet and Cardiodiabesity: A Systematic Review through Evidence-Based Answers to Key Clinical Questions.* Nutrients, *11*(3), 655. https://doi.org/10.3390/nu11030655

Davis, C., Bryan, J., Hodgson, J., & Murphy, K. (2015). *Definition of the Mediterranean Diet; a Literature Review.* Nutrients, *7*(11), 9139–9153. https://doi.org/10.3390/nu7115459

Bland, J. S., Minich, D. M., & Eck, B. M. (2017). *A Systems Medicine Approach: Translating Emerging Science into Individualized Wellness.* Advances in Medicine, *2017*, 1718957. https://doi.org/10.1155/2017/1718957

Lerman, R. H., Minich, D. M., Darland, G., Lamb, J. J., Schiltz, B., Babish, J. G., Bland, J. S., & Tripp, M. L. (2008). *Enhancement of a modified Mediterranean-style, low glycemic load diet with specific phytochemicals improves cardiometabolic risk factors in subjects with metabolic syndrome and hypercholesterolemia in a randomized trial.* Nutrition & Metabolism, *5*, 29. https://doi.org/10.1186/1743-7075-5-29

Weiskirchen, S., & Weiskirchen, R. (2016). *Resveratrol: How Much Wine Do You Have to Drink to Stay Healthy?* Advances in Nutrition *(Bethesda, Md.)* vol. 7,4 706-18. 15 Jul. doi:10.3945/an.115.011627

Snopek, L., Mlcek, J., Sochorova, L., Baron, M., Hlavacova, I., Jurikova, T., Kizek, R., Sedlackova, E., & Sochor, J. (2018). *Contribution of Red Wine Consumption to Human Health Protection. Molecules (Basel, Switzerland)*, *23*(7), 1684. https://doi.org/10.3390/molecules23071684

Emanuele, N. V., Swade, T. F., & Emanuele, M. A. (1998). *Consequences of alcohol use in diabetics.* Alcohol health and research world, *22*(3), 211–219.

Steiner, J. L., Crowell, K. T., & Lang, C. H. (2015). *Impact of Alcohol on Glycemic Control and Insulin Action.* Biomolecules, *5*(4), 2223–2246.

Velmourougane, K. (2016). *Impact of Organic and Conventional Systems of Coffee Farming on Soil Properties and Culturable Microbial Diversity.* Scientific Avol. 3604026. doi:10.1155/2016/3604026

Mekonen, S., Ambelu, A., & Spanoghe, P. (2015). *Effect of Household Coffee Processing on Pesticide Residues as a Means of Ensuring Consumers' Safety.* Journal of Agricultural and Food Chemistry, *63*(38), 8568–8573. https://doi.org/10.1021/acs.jafc.5b03327

Silverman, R. G. (2019). *Why Switch to Organic Coffee? Metagenics Blog*, 22 Feb

Butt, M. S., & Sultan, M. T. (2011). *Coffee and its consumption: benefits and risks. Critical Reviews in Food Science and Nutrition* vol. 51,4 363-73. doi:10.1080/10408390903586412

ActiveHerb. *Is Coffee Healthy? The Stimulating Answer According to TCM.*
Activeherb Blog, 5 Dec. 2019,

Institute of Medicine (US) Committee on Military Nutrition Research.
*Caffeine for the Sustainment of Mental Task Performance: Formulations for
Military Operations.* Washington (DC): National Academies Press (US);
2001. 2, Pharmacology of Caffeine.

McCusker, R. R., Fuehrlein, B., Goldberger, B. A., Gold, M. S., & Cone, E. J.
(2006). *Caffeine Content of Decaffeinated Coffee.* Journal of Analytical Toxicology,
30(8), 611–613. https://doi.org/10.1093/jat/30.8.611

Meinders, A-J. & Meinders, E. A. (2010). *How much water should we actually
drink?* Dutch Journal for Medicine vol. 154 A1757.

Popkin, B. M., D'Anci, K. E., & Rosenberg, I. H. (2010). *Water, hydration, and
health.* Nutrition Reviews, *68*(8), 439–458. https://doi.org/10.1111/j.1753-
4887.2010.00304.x

Armstrong, L. E., & Johnson, E. C. (2018). *Water Intake, Water Balance, and the
Elusive Daily Water Requirement.* Nutrients vol. 10,12 1928. 5 Dec., doi:10.3390/
nu10121928

Liska, D., Mah, E., Brisbois, T., Barrios, P. L., Baker, L. B., Spriet, L. L. (2019).
*Narrative Review of Hydration and Selected Health Outcomes in the General
Population,* Nutrients vol. 11,1 70. 1 Jan. doi:10.3390/nu11010070

*Report Sets Dietary Intake Levels for Water, Salt, and Potassium to Maintain Health
and Reduce Chronic Disease Risk. Nationalacademies.org,* The National Academies of
Sciences, Engineering, and Medicine, 11 Feb. 2004,

Meinders, A-J & Meinders, A. E., (2010) *Hoeveel water moeten we eigenlijk
drinken?" [How much water do we really need to drink?].* Nederlands tijdschrift voor
geneeskunde vol. 154 A1757.

CHAPTER 7: A RADIANT DAY

Gray A, & Threlkeld, R. J. (2019) *Nutritional Recommendations for Individuals with Diabetes.* [Updated Oct 13]. In: Feingold KR, Anawalt B, Boyce A, et al., editors. Endotext [Internet]. South Dartmouth (MA): MDText.com, Inc.; 2000-.

Ullrich I. H., & Albrink, M. J. *The effect of dietary fiber and other factors on insulin response: role in obesity.* J Environ Pathol Toxicol Oncol. 1985;5(6):137-155. https://pubmed.ncbi.nlm.nih.gov/2995635/

Fletcher, J. (2019) *Foods for Stabilizing Insulin and Blood Sugar Levels.* Medical News Today, MediLexicon International, 3 May,.https://www.medicalnewstoday.com/articles/323529#benefits-of-stabilizing-insulin-and-blood-sugar

Asif M. (2014). *The prevention and control the type-2 diabetes by changing lifestyle and dietary pattern.* Journal of Education and Health Promotion, 3, 1. https://doi.org/10.4103/2277-9531.127541

Childs, C. E., Calder, P. C., & Miles, E. A. (2019). *Diet and Immune Function.* Nutrients, 11(8), 1933. https://doi.org/10.3390/nu11081933

Calder, P. C. *Feeding the immune system.* Proc Nutr Soc. 2013;72(3):299-309. doi:10.1017/S0029665113001286

Corley, D. A., & Schuppan, D. (2015). *Food, the Immune System, and the Gastrointestinal Tract.* Gastroenterology, 148(6), 1083–1086. https://doi.org/10.1053/j.gastro.2015.03.043 https://www.ncbi.nlm.nih.gov/pmc/articles/PMC4409565/

Yan, Z., Zhong, Y., Duan, Y., Chen, Q., & Li, F. (2020). *Antioxidant mechanism of tea polyphenols and its impact on health benefits.* Animal Nutrition (Zhongguo xu mu shou yi xue hui), 6(2), 115–123. https://doi.org/10.1016/j.aninu.2020.01.001

Asif, N., Iqbal, R., & Nazir, C. F. (2017). *Human Immune System During Sleep.* American Journal of Clinical and Experimental Immunology 6, no. 6 92–96.

DiNicolantonio, J. J., O'Keefe, J. H., & Wilson, W. (2018). *Subclinical magnesium deficiency: a principal driver of cardiovascular disease and a public health crisis.* Open heart 5, no. 1 e000668. https://doi.org/10.1136/openhrt-2017-000668

Dhabhar F. S. *Effects of stress on immune function: the good, the bad, and the beautiful.* Immunol Res. 2014;58(2-3):193-210. doi:10.1007/s12026-014-8517-0 https://pubmed.ncbi.nlm.nih.gov/24798553/

Segerstrom S. C. (2007). *Stress, Energy, and Immunity: An Ecological View.* Current Directions in Psychological Science, 16(6), 326–330. https://doi.org/10.1111/j.1467-8721.2007.00522.x https://www.ncbi.nlm.nih.gov/pmc/articles/PMC2475648/

Chang C. Y., Ke, D. S., Chen, J. Y. *Essential Fatty Acids and Human Brain.* Acta Neurol Taiwan. 2009;18(4):231-241. https://pubmed.ncbi.nlm.nih.gov/20329590

Chianese, R., Coccurello, R., Viggiano, A., Scafuro, M., Fiore, M., Coppola, G., Operto, F. F., Fasano, S., Laye, S., Pierantoni, R., & Meccariello, R. (2018). *Impact of Dietary Fats on Brain Functions.* Current Neuropharmacology, 16(7), 1059–1085. https://doi.org/10.2174/1570159X15666171017102547

CHAPTER 8: SHOPPING LIST

Childs, C. E., Calder, P. C., & Miles, E. A. (2019). *Diet and Immune Function.* *Nutrients*, 11(8), 1933. https://doi.org/10.3390/nu11081933

Chen, Y., Michalak, M., & Agellon, L. B. (2018). *Importance of Nutrients and Nutrient Metabolism on Human Health.* The Yale Journal of Biology and Medicine, 91(2), 95–103.

Gómez-Pinilla F. (2008). *Brain foods: the effects of nutrients on brain function.* Nature Reviews. Neuroscience, 9(7), 568–578. https://doi.org/0.1038/nrn2421

Pizzorno J. (2014). *Mitochondria-Fundamental to Life and Health.* Integrative Medicine (Encinitas, Calif.), 13(2), 8–15.

Miller, V. J., Villamena, F. A., & Volek, J. S. (2018). *Nutritional Ketosis and Mitohormesis: Potential Implications for Mitochondrial Function and Human Health.* Journal of Nutrition and Metabolism, 2018, 5157645. https://doi.org/10.1155/2018/5157645

Sullivan, E. M., Pennington, E. R., Green, W. D., Beck, M. A., Brown, D. A., & Shaikh, S. R. (2018). *Mechanisms by Which Dietary Fatty Acids Regulate Mitochondrial Structure-Function in Health and Disease.* Advances in Nutrition (Bethesda, Md.), 9(3), 247–262. https://doi.org/10.1093/advances/nmy007

Kamangar, F., & Emadi, A. (2012). *Vitamin and mineral supplements: Do we really need them?* International Journal of Preventive Medicine, 3(3), 221–226.

Kaushal, M. J., & Magon, N. (2012). V*itamin D in Midlife: The sunrise vitamin in the sunset of life.* Journal of Mid-Life Health, 3(2), 97–99. https://doi.org/10.4103/0976-7800.104473

Nicolson G. L. (2014). *Mitochondrial Dysfunction and Chronic Disease: Treatment with Natural Supplements.* Integrative Medicine (Encinitas, Calif.), 13(4), 35–43.

Shen, L. R., Parnell, L. D., Ordovas, J. M., & Lai, C. Q. (2013). *Curcumin and aging.* BioFactors (Oxford, England), 39(1), 133–140. https://doi.org/10.1002/biof.1086

Bielak-Zmijewska, A., Grabowska, W., Ciolko, A., Bojko, A., Mosieniak, G., Bijoch, Ł., & Sikora, E. (2019). *The Role of Curcumin in the Modulation of Ageing.* International Journal of Molecular Sciences, 20(5), 1239. https://doi.org/10.3390/ijms20051239

Loria, K. (2019) *How to Choose Supplements Wisely.* Consumer Reports, 30 Oct.

Bailey R. L. (2020). C*urrent regulatory guidelines and resources to support research of dietary supplements in the United States.* Critical Reviews in Food Science and Nutrition, 60(2), 298–309. https://doi.org/10.1080/10408398.2018.1524364

Pandey, A., Tripathi, P., Pandey, R., Srivatava, R., & Goswami, S. (2011). *Alternative therapies useful in the management of diabetes: A systematic review.* Journal of Pharmacy & BioAllied Sciences, 3(4), 504–512. https://doi.org/10.4103/0975-7406.90103

Yin, J., Xing, H., & Ye, J. (2008). *Efficacy of berberine in patients with type 2 diabetes mellitus. Metabolism: Clinical and Experimental,* 57(5), 712–717. https://doi.org/10.1016/j.metabol.2008.01.013

Borkman, M., Chisholm, D. J., Furler, S. M., Storlien, L. H., Kraegen, E. W., Simons, L. A., & Chesterman, C. N. (1989). *Effects of Fish Oil Supplementation on Glucose and Lipid Metabolism in NIDDM.* Diabetes, 38(10), 1314–1319.https://doi.org/10.2337/diab.38.10.1314

Chauhan, S., Kodali, H., Noor, J., Ramteke, K., & Gawai, V. (2017). *Role of Omega-3 Fatty Acids on Lipid Profile in Diabetic Dyslipidaemia: Single Blind, Randomised Clinical Trial.* Journal of Clinical and Diagnostic Research : JCDR, 11(3), OC13–OC16. https://doi.org/10.7860/JCDR/2017/20628.9449

Mora, J. R., Iwata, M., & von Andrian, U. H. (2008). *Vitamin effects on the immune system: vitamins A and D take centre stage. Nature reviews. Immunology,* 8(9), 685–698. https://doi.org/10.1038/nri2378

Maggini, S., Pierre, A., & Calder, P. C. (2018). *Immune Function and Micronutrient Requirements Change over the Life Course.* Nutrients, 10(10), 1531. https://doi.org/10.3390/nu10101531

Carr, A. C., & Maggini, S. (2017). *Vitamin C and Immune Function.* Nutrients, 9(11), 1211. https://doi.org/10.3390/nu9111211

Wessels, I., Maywald, M., & Rink, L. (2017). *Zinc as a Gatekeeper of Immune Function.* Nutrients, 9(12), 1286. https://doi.org/10.3390/nu9121286

Bonaventura P, Benedetti G, Albarède F, Miossec P. *Zinc and Its Role in Immunity and Inflammation.* Autoimmun Rev. 2015;14(4):277-285. doi:10.1016/j.autrev.2014.11.008

Prasad A. S. (2008). *Zinc in Human Health: Effect of Zinc on Immune Cells.* Molecular medicine (Cambridge, Mass.), 14(5-6), 353–357. https://doi.org/10.2119/2008-00033.Prasad

Li, Y., Yao, J., Han, C., Yang, J., Chaudhry, M. T., Wang, S., Liu, H., & Yin, Y. (2016). *Quercetin, Inflammation and Immunity.* Nutrients, 8(3), 167. https://doi.org/10.3390/nu8030167

Malaguarnera L. (2019). *Influence of Resveratrol on the Immune Response.* Nutrients, 11(5), 946. https://doi.org/10.3390/nu11050946

Oliveira, A., Monteiro, V., Navegantes-Lima, K. C., Reis, J. F., Gomes, R. S., Rodrigues, D., Gaspar, S., & Monteiro, M. C. (2017). *Resveratrol Role in Autoimmune Disease-A Mini-Review.* Nutrients, 9(12), 1306. https://doi.org/10.3390/nu9121306

Suzuki, Y., Miyoshi, N., & Isemura, M. (2012). *Health-Promoting Effects of Green Tea.* Proceedings of the Japan Academy. Series B, Physical and Biological Sciences, 88(3), 88–101. https://doi.org/10.2183/pjab.88.88

Reygaert W. C. (2018). *Green Tea Catechins: Their Use in Treating and Preventing Infectious Diseases.* BioMed Research International, 2018, 9105261. https://doi.org/10.1155/2018/9105261

Grice, E. A., & Segre, J. A. (2011). *The Skin Microbiome.* Nature Reviews. Microbiology, 9(4), 244–253. https://doi.org/10.1038/nrmicro2537

Schagen, S. K., Zampeli, V. A., Makrantonaki, E., & Zouboulis, C. C. (2012). *Discovering the Link Between Nutrition and Skin Aging. Dermato-Endocrinology,* 4(3), 298–307. https://doi.org/10.4161/derm.22876

Panico, A., Serio, F., Bagordo, F., Grassi, T., Idolo, A., DE Giorgi, M., Guido, M., Congedo, M., & DE Donno, A. (2019). *Skin safety and health prevention: an overview of chemicals in cosmetic products.* Journal of Preventive Medicine and Hygiene, 60(1), E50–E57. https://doi.org/10.15167/2421-4248/jpmh2019.60.1.1080

CHAPTER 9: TRANSFORMATIONAL FOOD CLEANSE

Du, J., Zhu, M., Bao, H., Li, B., Dong, Y., Xiao, C., Zhang, G. Y., Henter, I., Rudorfer, M., & Vitiello, B. (2016). *The Role of Nutrients in Protecting Mitochondrial Function and Neurotransmitter Signaling: Implications for the Treatment of Depression, PTSD, and Suicidal Behaviors.* Critical reviews in food science and nutrition, 56(15), 2560–2578. https://doi.org/10.1080/10408398.2013.876960

Skin Exposures and Effects. Centers for Disease Control and Prevention, The National Institute for Occupational Safety and Health (NIOSH) , 2 July 2013. (No author)

Brown, H. S., Bishop, D. R., & Rowan, C. A. (1984). *The role of skin absorption as a route of exposure for volatile organic compounds (VOCs) in drinking water.* American Journal of Public Health, *74*(5), 479–484. https://doi.org/10.2105/ajph.74.5.479

CHAPTER 11: CHECKING IN AND STAYING ON TRACK

Scent Marketing for Hotels and Resorts: The Unexpected Advantage That Delivers the Best in Guest Experiences. ScentAir. (No author)

Scent HalO Light, *ScentAndrea* LLC, (No author)

Herz, R. (2008) *Buying by the Nose. Adweek,* Adweek, 21 Jan.

Cuda, G. (2010). *Marketers Know It's Hard to Resist Foods When You're Tempted by Scents: Fighting Fat.* Cleveland, Advance Local Media LLC, 6 Apr.

Leech, J. (2020) *Lemon Water 101: What Are the Benefits of Drinking It?* Medical News Today, MediLexicon International,14 May www.medicalnewstoday.com/articles/318662#benefits.

Larsen, N., Bussolo de Souza, C., Krych, L., Barbosa Cahú, T., Wiese, M., Kot, W., Hansen, K. M., Blennow, A., Venema, K., & Jespersen, L. (2019). *Potential of Pectins to • Beneficially Modulate the Gut Microbiota Depends on Their Structural Properties. frontiers in Microbiology, 10,* 223. https://doi.org/10.3389/fmicb.2019.00223

ADAPTOGEN GLOSSARY

Panda, A. K., & Swain, K. C. (2011). *Traditional uses and medicinal potential of Cordyceps sinensis of Sikkim. Journal of Ayurveda and Integrative Medicine* vol. 2,1 9-13. doi:10.4103/0975-9476.78183

Lee, C. C., Lee, Y. L., Wang, C. N., Tsai, H. C., Chiu, C. L., Liu, L. F., Lin, H. Y., & Wu, R. (2016). *Polygonum multiflorum Decreases Airway Allergic Symptoms in a Murine Model of Asthma.* The American Journal of Chinese Medicine, 44(1), 133–147. https://doi.org/10.1142/S0192415X16500099

Faerman, J. (2019) T*his Ancient Herb Is Prized For Its Ability to Expand Intuition and Extend Lifespan.* Conscious Lifestyle Magazine, 22 Apr.

Chong, P. S., Fung, M. L., Wong, K. H., & Lim, L. W. (2019). *Therapeutic Potential of Hericium erinaceus for Depressive Disorder.* International Journal of Molecular Sciences, 21(1), 163. https://doi.org/10.3390/ijms21010163

Chacko, S. M., Thambi, P. T., Kuttan, R., & Nishigaki, I. (2010). *Beneficial Effects of Green Tea: A Literature Review.* Chinese Medicine, 5, 13. https://doi.org/10.1186/1749-8546-5-13

Unno, K., Furushima, D., Hamamoto, S., Iguchi, K., Yamada, H., Morita, A., Horie, H., & Nakamura, Y. (2018). *Stress-Reducing Function of Matcha Green Tea in Animal Experiments and Clinical Trials.* Nutrients, 10(10), 1468. https://doi.org/10.3390/nu10101468

Dietz, C., Dekker, M., & Piqueras-Fiszman, B. (2017). *An intervention study on the effect of matcha tea, in drink and snack bar formats, on mood and cognitive performance.* Food research international (Ottawa, Ont.), 99(Pt 1), 72–83. https://doi.org/10.1016/j.foodres.2017.05.002

Suzuki, Y., Miyoshi, N., & Isemura, M. (2012). *Health-promoting effects of green tea.* Proceedings of the Japan Academy. Series B, Physical and Biological Sciences, 88(3), 88–101. https://doi.org/10.2183/pjab.88.88

Bonuccelli, G., Sotgia, F., & Lisanti, M. P. (2018). *Matcha green tea (MGT) inhibits the propagation of cancer stem cells (CSCs), by targeting mitochondrial metabolism, glycolysis and multiple cell signalling pathways.* Aging, 10(8), 1867–1883. https://doi.org/10.18632/aging.101483

Suresh, S., Prithiviraj, E., Lakshmi, N. V., Ganesh, M. K., Ganesh, L., & Prakash, S. (2013). *Effect of Mucuna pruriens (Linn.) on mitochondrial dysfunction and DNA damage in epididymal sperm of streptozotocin induced diabetic rat.* Journal of Ethnopharmacology, 145(1), 32–41. https://doi.org/10.1016/j.jep.2012.10.030

Shukla, K. K., Mahdi, A. A., Ahmad, M. K., Jaiswar, S. P., Shankwar, S. N., & Tiwari, S. C. (2010). *Mucuna pruriens Reduces Stress and Improves the Quality of Semen in Infertile Men. Evidence-based complementary and alternative medicine : eCAM,* 7(1), 137–144. https://doi.org/10.1093/ecam/nem171

Rana, D. G., & Galani, V. J. (2014). *Dopamine mediated antidepressant effect of Mucuna pruriens seeds in various experimental models of depression.* Ayu vol. 35,1 90-7. doi:10.4103/0974-8520.141949

Katzenschlager, R., Evans, A., Manson, A., Patsalos, P. N., Ratnaraj, N., Watt, H., Timmermann, L., Van der Giessen, R., & Lees, A. J. (2004). *Mucuna pruriens in Parkinson's disease: a double blind clinical and pharmacological study. Journal of Neurology, Neurosurgery, and Psychiatry,* 75(12), 1672–1677. https://doi.org/10.1136/jnnp.2003.028761

Chiu H. F., Hsiao S. C., Lu Y. Y., Han Y. C., Shen Y. C., Venkatakrishna K., & Wang, C. K. (2017) *Efficacy of Protein Rich Pearl Powder on Antioxidant Status in a Randomized Placebo-Controlled Trial. Journal of Food and Drug Analysis,* Elsevier, 13 June

Bai, J. (2015) *Electrospun Composites of PHBV/Pearl Powder for Bone Repairing. Science Direct,* RELX, Aug.

Faerman, J. (2020) *The Health Benefits of Pearl Powder: Superfood from the Sea. Conscious Lifestyle Magazine,* 22 Jan., www.consciouslifestylemag.com/pearl-powder-benefits/.

Wachtel-Galor S, Yuen J, Buswell J. A., Benzie I. F-F. (2011) Ganoderma lucidum (Lingzhi or Reishi): A Medicinal Mushroom. In: Benzie I. F-F, Wachtel-Galor S, editors. *Herbal Medicine: Biomolecular and Clinical Aspects.* 2nd edition. Boca Raton (FL): CRC Press/Taylor & Francis; Chapter 9.

Szopa, A., Ekiert, R., & Ekiert, H. (2017). *Current knowledge of Schisandra chinensis (Turcz.) Baill. (Chinese magnolia vine) as a medicinal plant species: a review on the bioactive components, pharmacological properties, analytical and biotechnological studies.* Phytochemistry reviews : proceedings of the Phytochemical Society of Europe, 16(2), 195–218. https://doi.org/10.1007/s11101-016-9470-4

Alok, S., Jain, S. K., Verma, A., Kumar, M., Mahor, A., & Sabharwal, M. (2013). *Plant profile, phytochemistry and pharmacology of Asparagus racemosus (Shatavari): A review.* Asian Pacific Journal of Tropical Disease, 3(3), 242–251. https://doi.org/10.1016/S2222-1808(13)60049-3

CPSIA information can be obtained
at www.ICGtesting.com
Printed in the USA
JSHW030834071120
9397JS00002B/6

9 781734 956320